Carol Braga.

San Francisco, 1972

CYTOPATHOLOGY *of*
FEMALE GENITAL TRACT NEOPLASMS

of FEMALE

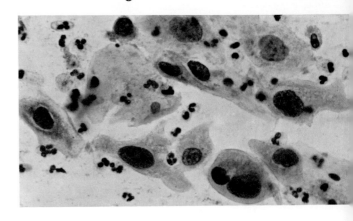

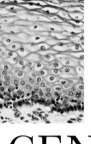

CYTOPATHOLOGY
GENITAL TRACT
NEOPLASMS

by

DUANE N. TWEEDDALE, M. D.

*Department of Pathology, St. Elizabeth Hospital
and Medical Center, Dayton Ohio*

and

LOUIS D. DUBILIER, M. D.

*Pathology and Cytology Laboratory and
Central Baptist Hospital;
Clinical Assistant Professor of Pathology,
University of Kentucky College of Medicine, Lexington, Kentucky*

35 EAST WACKER DRIVE • CHICAGO

YEAR BOOK MEDICAL PUBLISHERS • INC.

Library of Congress Catalog Card Number: 74-165965

International Standard Book Number: 0-8151-8890-0

To my ELSIE
who gave inspiration in the past
and strength for the future

D.N.T.

Preface

ALMOST EVERY BOOK serves a useful purpose, whether it be for the satisfaction of the author or the gratification of the reader. In compiling this volume, we have attained the former by recording certain ideas and concepts in the field of cytology that we believe are valuable. The book has ample references but does not pretend to be a compendium of all available information. The field of cytology has become so broad in such a short time that its full context could not be covered in a single or even in several volumes. Investigators have so extended the range of cytologic interpretation that, for example, one is seldom content merely to suggest the probability of the existence of cancer. Indeed, a cancer diagnosis is often so refined that it not only delineates the specific cell type but indicates whether a malignant lesion is in situ or invasive. In addition, the modern cytologist usually understands and applies practically, where feasible, the principles of chromosome analysis, cytochemistry, electron microscopy, labeling studies, microspectrophotometry, computer analysis, mensuration by automated means, Coulter counter and hormonocytologic studies. It is our purpose to supply the reader with practical information directed primarily to the cytologic diagnosis of gynecologic cancer. Comparison of these findings with cytologic observations suggesting or simulating malignant neoplasia is included in chapters dealing primarily with changes due to inflammation, repair, degeneration and radiation. Sections dealing with microspectrophotometric and computer application are intended to bridge the gap between what is now research and what might be tomorrow's reality. Chromosome studies, labeling and electron microscopy are similarly considered. Despite future advances, the cytotechnologist will always play an important role in cytodiagnosis. No matter how advanced, machines do not have a "brain" but reflect primarily the imagination and intelligence of the user. For example, despite the automation of chemical, hematologic, coagulation and other routine clinical laboratory procedures, there is still a serious shortage of medical technologists.

We hope that technology students, graduate technologists, resident physicians, pathologists, gynecologists and other physicians and scientists interested in the cytologic diagnosis of female genital tract neoplasms will find this book valuable, both as a means of improving the precision of their diagnoses and as a reference source.

Acknowledgments

There are many people to whom we are indebted for their varied contributions to this book. Very special thanks go to all the cytotechnologists who through the years have given their time and energies to make this work possible. Mrs. Marjorie Laslie Holt, CT (ASCP), spent many dedicated hours maintaining special files so that we could extract cases of particular interest. Mrs. Mary Jane Fields Henderson, CT (ASCP), formerly our chief technologist, helped create a dynamic cytology section in a new medical school.

The following people participated in various research projects, the data from which is included throughout the book: Mrs. Sara Whitehouse Elam, CT (ASCP); Miss Elaine Kington; Mrs. Sandra Langenback, CT (ASCP); Mrs. Sandra Moore Mills; Earl Nelson, M.D.; Eula Jean Noble, CT (ASCP); William Offutt, M.D.; Charles Stephens, M.D.; and Carl Watson, M.D. The contribution of each was invaluable.

Our clinical colleagues, especially those from the Department of Obstetrics and Gynecology, have faithfully supported and encouraged our cytology program. Dr. John W. Greene, chairman of the Department of Obstetrics and Gynecology, and Dr. John W. Roddick, Jr., have been our closest allies.

Our secretarial staff, Mrs. Ted Herbert, Miss Shirley Calvert and Mrs. Phillip Lykins, have provided us with patient assistance.

We would be remiss if we forgot to express our gratitude to Year Book Medical Publishers for their patience and understanding.

Within the Department of Pathology, all of our colleagues have offered many constructive criticisms. To our special critic, Herbert Braunstein, M.D., we cannot find proper words to express our heartfelt thanks. In no way is he responsible for imperfections that may be detected. Finally, we want to thank W. B. "Pete" Stewart, M.D., our department chairman, for his encouragement and for creating available time to pursue this project.

D.N.T.
L.D.D.

Table of Contents

CHAPTER 1

History

THE USE OF CYTOLOGIC study to diagnose malignancy dates back to the 19th century. Most of the earlier workers concentrated on microscopic examination of sputum. In 1847, Pouchet[16] examined vaginal secretions while studying the problem of whether spontaneous ovulation occurs in animals and man. He observed epithelial plaques in the vagina during menstruation and also noted gross changes in vaginal secretions. It is not certain whether actual microscopic examination was done on the secretions as he did not detail his methodology. As late as 1869,[11] the value of vaginal cytology in the diagnosis of gynecologic malignancy was denied. The major interest in gynecologic cellular examination continued to be the study of hormonal changes, earlier in the guinea pig and rat, and later in humans.[10] Papanicolaou[15] discussed the potential value of vaginal smears as an aid in the diagnosis of uterine cancer with Dr. James Ewing in 1925. Because of limitations in both cytologic and histopathologic knowledge, he did not realize fully that asymptomatic cervical cancer could be diagnosed by such means. In fact, Broders[2] did not coin the term carcinoma in situ until 1932, although the condition had been described years earlier. On April 11, 1928, Dr. Aurel A. Babes[1] published a monumental communication in *La Presse Médicale* entitled, "Diagnosis of Cancer of the Uterine Cervix by Smears." His material was collected by a platinum loop, fixed in methyl alcohol and stained with the Giemsa method. He detailed and illustrated characteristics of malignant cells, indicated the existence of carcinoma in situ and stated that the diagnosis of cervical cancer could be made at an early stage by the smear technique. His work had been first presented to the Society of Gynecology of Bucharest on January 23, 1927, and again on April 10, 1927. Almost simultaneously, Papanicolaou,[8] at the Third Race Betterment Conference held January 2–6, 1928, at Battle Creek, Michigan, reported independently the occurrence of malignant cells as seen by cytology. His paper entitled "New Cancer Diagnosis" described his technique, which utilized a small pipette to remove vaginal fluid, and indicated cytologic characteristics of malignant cells. His foresight was reflected by the following quote:

"We have a better understanding of the situation in a cancer case, and we may have some help in analyzing the cancer problem in the future. In fact, I think this work will be carried a little further, and that analogous methods may be applied in the recognition of cancers in other organs. I think that some such method can be, and will be, developed in the future."

Thirteen years later, in collaboration with H. F. Traut, he published "Diagnostic Value of Vaginal Smears in Carcinoma of the Uterus."[13] They not only described cellular changes in invasive cervical carcinoma and endometrial adenocarcinoma but indicated the possibility of a positive cytodiagnosis in early stages of those diseases. A further contribution in 1943[14] recorded two instances of early carcinoma of the cervix and endometrium detected initially by cytologic means. That same year they published a 48-page monograph, entitled "Diagnosis of Uterine Cancer by the Vaginal Smear," that included twelve color plates.[15] The readers will be interested in an excellent biography of the late Dr. Papanicolaou by Leopold G. Koss.[7]

Through support by the American Cancer Society and the United States Public Health Service, expansion and corroboration of the value of cytology in the early diagnosis of uterine malignancy, primarily cervical, was established. The mass survey projects started in 1952 eventually revealed the high incidence of unsuspected cervical cancer, further establishing a role of cytology in medicine.[5, 6] In the course of such studies, up to 83% of white women and 69% of Negro women from a select area had a vaginal cytologic examination.[6] For the most part, vaginal cytologic diagnosis still was in embryonic stages in the early 1950's. This was the natural result of a technique requiring time and experience to master, both for the technologist and cytopathologist, as well as a necessary period in which the practicing physician gained understanding of and confidence in the method. Schools of cytotechnology were established and registry examinations were first administered in 1957 by the American Society of Clinical Pathologists. Cytology became part of the American Board of Pathology examination in 1962. Many workers promoted cytology through a plethora of articles in the 1950's and 1960's. *Acta Cytologica*, a journal devoted to cytology, published its first issue in 1956. The sum total of the above efforts has saved tens of thousands of lives annually. As an important bonus, cytology has led to the most intense study to date on the genesis of early cancer.

Despite the now unquestioned merit of the vaginal smear in the early diagnosis of cervical cancer, it is discouraging that only about 15% of all women over the age of 20 in the United States had a Papanicolaou smear examined in 1963.[4, 17] Thus, there remains a vast reservoir of women with cervical cancer who may die because a simple, inexpensive technique has not been applied. We feel that the smear examination is an integral part of an adequate physical examination. Indeed, it has been suggested that, in our insurance-conscious population, a cytologic examination is the cheapest insurance available.[3]

REFERENCES

1. Babes, A.: Diagnosis of cancer of the uterine cervix by smears, Presse méd. 36:451, 1928; abstracted by Douglas, L. D.: Acta cytol. 11:217, 1967.
2. Broders, A. C.: Carcinoma in situ contrasted with benign penetrating epithelium, J.A.M.A. 99:1670, 1932.
3. Christopherson, W. M.: The control of cervix cancer, Acta cytol. 10:6, 1966.
4. Christopherson, W. M., and Watanabe, G.: A survey of cytopathology facilities in the United States, Bull. Coll. Am. Pathologists, June, 1965, p. 108.
5. Erickson, C. C., et al.: Preliminary report of 20,000 women studied by the vaginal smear technique in a general population cancer screening project, Proc. Am. Assoc. Cancer Res. (abstract) 1:14, April, 1953.
6. Kashgarian, M., et al.: A survey of public awareness of uterine cytology in Memphis-Shelby County, Acta cytol. 10:11, 1966.
7. Koss, L. G.: George N. Papanicolaou (1883–1962), Acta cytol. 7:143, 1963.
8. Papanicolaou, G. N.: Proc. of the Third Race Betterment Conference, Battle Creek, Mich., Jan. 2–6, 1928, p. 528.
9. Papanicolaou, G. N.: The sexual cycle in the human female as revealed by vaginal smears, Am. J. Anat. 52:519, 1933.
10. Papanicolaou, G. N.: A general survey of the vaginal smear and its use in research and diagnosis, Am. J. Obst. & Gynec. 51:316, 1946.
11. Papanicolaou, G. N.: A survey of the actualities and potentialities of exfoliative cytology in cancer diagnosis, Am. Int. Med. 31:661, 1949.
12. Papanicolaou, G. N.: Historical development of cytology as a tool in clinical medicine and in cancer research, Acta Un. Int. Cancer, 14:249, 1958.
13. Papanicolaou, G. N., and Traut, H. G.: The diagnostic value of vaginal smears in carcinoma of the uterus, Am. J. Obst. & Gynec. 42:193, 1941.
14. Papanicolaou, G. N., and Traut, H. G.: The demonstration of malignant cells in vaginal smears and its relation to the diagnosis of carcinoma of the uterus, New York J. Med. 43:767, 1943.
15. Papanicolaou, G. N., and Traut, H. G.: Diagnosis of Uterine Cancer by the Vaginal Smear (New York: The Commonwealth Fund, 1943).
16. Pouchet, F. A.: Theórie Positive de l'Ovulation Spontanée et de la Fécondation des Mammifères et de l'Espèc Humaine, Basée Sur l'Observation de Toute la Série Animale (Paris: J. B. Baillière et fils, 1847), with an atlas with 20 colored plates, p. 245.
17. The Gallup Organization, Inc.: The Public's Awareness and Use of Cancer Detection Tests (Princeton, N. J., 1964).
18. Wied, G. L.: Pap test or Babes method (Editorial), Acta cytol. 8:173, 1964.

CHAPTER 2

Diagnostic Value of Cervicovaginal Cytology

THE USE OF VAGINAL cytology is predicated on the premise that lesions diagnosed by this method actually are early stages in the genesis of malignancy. The logical result of their ablation would be to prevent progression to later stages of cervical or endometrial cancer. More specifically, there is much corroborative evidence to indicate that carcinoma in situ of the cervix, a term coined by Broders in 1932[3, 26] but described earlier under a variety of names, is a precursor of invasive cancer.[26, 29] The evidence has been of a statistical or morphologic nature; the latter will be discussed in a subsequent chapter. Because of the recognized importance of diagnosing cervical cancer early, the present discussion stresses the value of vaginal cytology. This will be approached from the viewpoint of:

1. Incidence of positive cytologic diagnoses in initial screening.
2. Incidence of positive cytologic diagnoses in subsequent screenings.
3. Effect of the above on the incidence of invasive cervical cancer.
4. Prevalence of dysplasia in initially and rescreened populations.
5. The role of cytodiagnosis in adenocarcinoma of the cervix and endometrium.
6. Cytology during pregnancy.
7. Teenage cytology.

Since the pick-up rate for cervical cancer is dependent on such factors as socioeconomic status, race, age, parity and religion, the statistical data of any series must be interpreted with care, acknowledging potential peculiarities or circumstances surrounding a particular locale.

Incidence of Positive Cytologic Diagnoses in Initial Screening

Large collected series are heavily weighted by cases from community surveys. They give a good cross-section of a particular population, being influenced primarily by the population distribution related to socioeconomic status. Other series may be quite selective. For example, Papanicolaou's[39] first series of 3,014 women resulted in the diagnosis of 7 cases of in situ carcinoma (0.23%) and of 120 cases of invasive carcinoma (4%). The high per cent of invasive lesions was the result of a select group of women attending that cancer diagnostic clinic. By contrast, analysis of initial screenings, gleaned mainly from community or area surveys,[9, 18, 31, 36, 51, 55, 58] reveals that slightly over 1% will be found to have cervical carcinoma, of which the invasive lesions outnumber in situ carcinomas (0.577% vs. 0.487%). To emphasize the strong modifying factor of the socioeconomic status of those examined, Ludin, *et al.*,[35] observed that the annual incidence rates for cervical cancer were 54.3 per 100,000 whites. Others[50] have noted surprisingly similar results. Caucasians living in a low socioeconomic area also have a similarly high incidence of cervical cancer. This has been our experience in studying cervical cancer among women living in severely depressed economic areas of Appalachia. For example, our ratio of cervical carcinoma to endometrial carcinoma is about 7.5:1. Because of neglect prevalent among those of low socioeconomic levels, cervical neoplasia in whites, when compared with Negroes, ordinarily will be found in earlier stages of genesis when discovered initially.[35, 50] In contrast, a large series from a private clinic revealed that 90% of cervical squamous carcinomas were in situ.[15] In addition, the factors of early marriage (and coitus) and multiparity, usually paralleling a low socioeconomic status, will be found associated with those women having more cervical cancer than a control population.[1, 8, 11, 12, 20, 21, 47, 53]

Incidence of Positive Cytologic Diagnoses in Subsequent Screenings

Marshall[36] noted in the course of an active screening program over a 6-year period (1958–1963) that the total number of cases of cervical carcinoma confirmed by biopsy dropped from 0.71% to 0.15%. The incidence drop was attributed to a progressive screening-out process in which approximately 60% of the women were screened at least twice. The decline in the incidence of invasive cervical carcinoma was striking, opposed to a fairly stable rate for those of in situ nature. Sprunt and Berton[50] found 2.8 cervical carcinomas per 1,000 white women among 73,422 screened for the first time, and a corresponding 5.6 per 1,000 nonwhite women among 34,785 screened. Of the total of 108,207 women, 0.38% had invasive cervical cancer and 0.38% had carcinoma in situ. The second screening resulted in 0.2 cervical cancers per 1,000 white women among 20,783 screened, and 0.6 per 1,000 nonwhite women among 11,955 screenings. Of the total of 32,738 women, 0.25% had invasive cervical cancer and 0.04% had carcinoma in situ. They believed that the incidence drop with a rescreening is the result of the natural history of the cancer. Christopherson, *et al.*[9] observed an initial incidence of 2.8 per 1,000 women with invasive cervical carcinoma and 3.7 women per 1,000 with carcinoma in situ among 66,043 screened. By the third annual screening of 9,518 women, only 0.11 per 1,000 had invasive cervical cancer and 0.53 per 1,000 had carcinoma in situ. They believed "that repeated examinations at yearly intervals would virtually eliminate cervical cancer as a major cause of death in our female population." Others[15] recording similar findings feel that repeat annual smears "weed out" cases of invasive cervical carcinoma from the test population. Bryans, *et al.*[4] saw an almost tenfold increase in invasive cervical carcinoma among those not previously screened when compared with those who had annual smear studies.

Effect of Vaginal Cytologic Examination on the Pattern of Invasive Cervical Carcinoma

The above studies have been unanimous with respect to the efficacy of cytologic screening to diagnose cervical carcinoma. In a population that has been screened adequately, and especially rescreened, as indicated, the subsequent pick-up rate of cervical carcinoma has been reduced, often dramatically. That is true mainly of invasive carcinoma, but also to a lesser degree for carcinoma in situ. Regarding the occurrence of invasive cervical carcinoma in a screened population, certain important facts emerge.[2, 4, 22, 52] The result of an active screening program is a progressive decrease in the number of women with invasive cervical cancers. The invasive cancers that have been cytologically identified in these circumstances generally are found in earlier stages.[31, 35, 52] For example, Stevenson, *et al,*[52] noted that the incidence of stage I and II carcinomas increased from 56% to 75% over a 12-year period, whereas stage III and IV lesions decreased from 44% to 25% during that same period.

However, the sum total of the value of screening programs should be reflected in mortality statistics of a screened community. Christopherson[6] noted a gradual decline in reported mortality statistics from cervical cancer in Jefferson County, Kentucky. The drop was not precipitous, but there are some factors possibly accounting for that finding. First, a few cases may have been women who were relatively long survivors of a disease diagnosed in the early days of cytologic experience. Second, and most likely of greater importance, are the women who had not been screened in the population. Many of them may have been indigent, as that group is often the most difficult to get to co-operate and is the one most likely to get cervical carcinoma. Added factors may be false negative diagnoses in the face of invasive carcinoma, and a transient population.

Prevalence of Dysplasia in Initially Screened and Rescreened Populations

The prevalence of dysplasia is variable, having been reported from 0.13% to 3.8% of selected series. Reagan[40] believes that it occurs in 0.8% of all women, although he found 6.2% of a group of pregnant patients from a charity clinic to have that abnormality.[43] Among 2,417 pregnant women seen at our institution, 26 (1.1%) had dysplasia. Despite that finding, the lesion does seem to be distinctly more frequent among pregnant females. The variable incidences are undoubtedly reflective of the population screened, for, if a series contains a large number of pregnant women, the incidence may be overwhelmingly high.[43] In common with in situ carcinoma, dysplasia has a high incidence in the lower socioeconomic groups, being at least twice that of a routinely screened population in Christopherson's studies.[7,9] In contrast, if a predominately older group of women is screened, there will be a lower incidence of dysplasia, a reflection of the mean age of 34 years at detection of that lesion.[41]

Of populations rescreened, dysplasia has been discovered with equal or slightly decreased frequency as the original screening. In contrast, squamous cell epithelioma in situ has demonstrated a more marked decrease in incidence.[9,18] What is the significance of such a finding? Possibly, it is a reflection of ablation of a precursor to in situ cancer and the subsequent occurrence of a constant number of new cases with dysplasia, most remaining static but a few progressing to cancer.

The Role of Cytodiagnosis in Adenocarcinoma of the Cervix and Endometrium

It is axiomatic in cytology that the accuracy and pick-up rate, in general, is inversely proportional to the distance that abnormal cells have to travel before collection. For example, cytodetection of pulmonary neoplasms is considerably poorer than is that of the cervix, as the latter site lends ready anatomic availability. When contrasting cytodetection of cervical and endometrial adenocarcinoma, it is readily apparent that the former area yields a much higher incidence of symptomatic and asymptomatic lesions. In fact, Koss and Durfee identified only one case of endometrial carcinoma in screening 5,000 asymptomatic patients.[34] There are several reasons why cervical and vaginal smears fail to reveal endometrial cancer.[23] The endometrial cancer cells travel a modest distance and may degenerate; cervical stenosis is not uncommon in the postmenopause; and cell exfoliation does not approach that seen from cervical neoplasia. In general, 50%–75% of all females with endometrial adenocarcinoma are detected by routine cervical cytologic studies.[10, 13, 42] Unfortunately, in only a small number of patients (8%–14%),[13, 42] abnormal cells seen in cytologic smears will be the sole evidence for further investigation and subsequent tissue diagnosis of endometrial adenocarcinoma. Thus, most will be symptomatic, usually with vaginal bleeding, and already are candidates for definitive diagnostic studies such as curettage. The total number of cases of endometrial adenocarcinoma also will be considerably fewer than those of squamous carcinoma of the cervix. There is evidence indicating that less endometrial carcinoma is to be expected in lower socioeconomic groups.[10] It is still an unusual disease before 40 years of age, so that pick-up rate is influenced by age distribution among screened patients. Some authors[24] have indicated that the ratio of invasive cervical cancer to endometrial cancer is coming closer to 1:1 because of the influence of Papanicolaou smears in detecting in situ cancers and thereby preventing the invasive sequel. Notwithstanding, it still seems doubtful whether enough asymptomatic endometrial cancers can be detected by routine methods to justify time and expense (for that purpose alone).[15]

Some investigators have advocated endometrial aspiration smears to diagnose carcinoma of the fundus, indicating a high degree of accuracy.[23, 42] Yet, all the established indications for that procedure refer to abnormal bleeding.[23] Thus, the criteria for detection of clinically unsuspected disease still are not met.

The diagnosis of endocervical adenocarcinoma by cytologic means is more practical than it is for endometrial carcinoma. Fewer endocervical neoplasms will be seen, however, as only 5% of cervical malignancies are adenocarcinoma.[25] In contrast to the endometrium, the cervical area is more amenable to direct removal and examination of cellular elements. Indeed, the cytologic recognition of adenocarcinoma of the cervix is about 90%,[13, 42] of which around 40% will be asymptomatic. The pick-up rate, and especially identification of asymptomatic lesions, is intermediate between that of adenocarcinoma of the endometrium and squamous cell carcinoma of the cervix. The practicality is unquestioned because of detection of a large number of asymptomatic cases. There are a number of cases in recent literature of endocervical adenocarcinoma in situ or of very early adenocarcinoma diagnosed primarily by cytology.[37]

Cytology During Pregnancy

There is no laboratory contraindication to obtaining cervical smears in the pregnant female. It is urged that every pregnant woman have a cytologic examination unless serious clinical contraindications exist, i.e., protruding bag of waters. Because cervical cancer is unusual in those who have not had multiple births, it may be possible to detect that neoplasm in its very early stage of genesis during repeat visits to the obstetrician. Again, it is the indigent patient who makes up the high-risk group.[49] The average age at which in situ cancer is detected in the pregnant patient has been noted to be 27 years; this falls substantially below the peak incidence of in situ cervical cancer in the general population and even more so of the invasive counterpart.[27] In one composite report, 0.35% of all pregnant females had cervical carcinoma in pregnancy (in situ and invasive).[54] This, of course, is considerably more than half as frequent as the general population, most of whom are not pregnant. Of all patients with carcinoma in situ, at least one in six will be pregnant.[28] In different reports of carcinoma in situ in pregnant women, the incidence of that disease varied from 0.03% to 0.5%, and it is reasonable to conclude that about 0.2%–0.3% of all pregnant women will have in situ carcinoma. In general, those with in situ carcinoma during pregnancy will be in a slightly older age bracket than the usual pregnant patient.[54]

A much smaller number of pregnant women will have invasive carcinoma than in situ carcinoma, the ratio varying from 1:4 to 0:28.[16, 17, 30, 33, 38, 44, 45, 48, 54, 57] From 0.14% to 0.01% will have invasive malignancy.[45] Those patients will account for 0.2% to 5.0% of total cervical carcinomas.[45, 56] Since the majority will be in an early stage, the cytologist has an added responsibility for accurate diagnosis so that therapy can be instituted promptly.

The high incidence of dysplasia during pregnancy has been indicated in a previous section. The biologic behavior is discussed in detail in another chapter.

Teenage Cytology

It is generally accepted that the peak incidence of in situ cervical cancer occurs at age 38, 10 years earlier than its invasive counterpart. While uncommon, 6%–14% of invasive cervical cancers may occur in the third decade.[5, 19, 46] If one accepts that in situ cancer, with its fairly long latent period, is a precursor of the invasive lesion, it should not be surprising that atypical (dysplastic) changes, or intraepithelial carcinomas, can be seen in teenagers. Ferguson[19] found smears positive for cancer or dysplasia in patients as young as 14 years of age; most of the girls presenting abnormal findings were Negro (4:1). Of ten girls with in situ carcinoma, two were 16 years of age. Those with dysplasia outnumbered the in situ cases by at least 2:1. Ferguson's material was gleaned from 1,500 women with positive smears of which 77 (0.5%) were 19 years or younger. Unfortunately, many were not biopsied and admittedly were from a select group in whom the incidence of pregnancies was high and sexual promiscuity and infection common.[14, 19] Kaufman, et al.[32] studied 1,199 teenage patients on whom cytology was done. They found three cases of dysplasia and two of in situ carcinoma, a pick-up rate of 0.16% for in situ epithelioma. The question of who should have a vaginal smear is a logical sequel to the fact that in situ and, very rarely, invasive carcinoma may occur before 20 years of age. The value of cytology in the third decade is unquestioned because of the occurrence of cervical carcinoma, usually in situ, in that age period.[5] We believe that any woman who has a pelvic examination deserves to have a smear study as an essential part of a complete physical examination. Obviously, women who are not virgins, and especially those with onset of intercourse early in life, are prime candidates for cytodetection of neoplasia.[35]

REFERENCES

1. Boyd, J. T., and Doll, R.: A study of the aetiology of carcinoma of the cervix uteri, Brit. J. Cancer 18:419, 1964.
2. Boyes, D. A., Fidler, H. K., and Lock, D. R.: Significance of in situ carcinoma of the uterine cervix, Brit. M. J. 5273:203, 1962.
3. Broders, A. C.: Carcinoma in situ contrasted with benign penetrating epithelium, Collect. Papers Mayo Clin. 24:1111, 1932.
4. Bryans, F. E., Boyes, D. A., and Fidler, H. K.: The influence of a cytological screening program upon the incidence of invasive squamous cell carcinoma of the cervix in British Columbia, Am. J. Obst. & Gynec. 88:898, 1964.
5. Cavanagh, D., McLeod, A. G. W., and Ferguson, J., II: Carcinoma of the cervix among women in their twenties. A 14% prevalence deserves our respect, J.A.M.A. 195:834, 1966.
6. Christopherson, W. M.: The control of cervix cancer, Acta cytol. 10:6, 1966.
7. Christopherson, W. M., and Parker, J. E.: A study of the relative frequency of carcinoma of the cervix in the Negro, Cancer 13:711, 1960.
8. Christopherson, W. M., and Parker, J. E.: Relation of cervical cancer to early marriage and childbearing, New England J. Med. 273:235, 1965.
9. Christopherson, W. M., Parker, J. E., and Drye, J. C.: Control of cervical cancer, preliminary report on community program, J.A.M.A. 182:179, 1962.
10. Christopherson, W. M., et al.: A ten-year study of endometrial carcinoma in Louisville, Kentucky, Cancer 18:554, 1965.
11. Clemmesen, J., and Nielsen, A.: The social distribution of cancer in Copenhagen, 1943–1947, Brit. J. Cancer 5:159, 1951.
12. Cohart, E. M.: Socioeconomic distribution of cancer of the female sex organs in New Haven, Cancer 8:34, 1955.
13. Coleman, S. A., Rube, I. F., and Erickson, C. C.: Cytologic detection of adenocarcinoma of the uterus in a mass screening project, Am. J. Obst. & Gynec. 92:472, 1965.
14. Craig, J. M.: Letter to the Editor, J.A.M.A. 180:177, 1962.
15. Dahlin, D. C., et al.: Smears in the detection of preclinical carcinoma of the uterine cervix: further studies with emphasis on the significance of the negative "repeats," Surg. Gynec. & Obst. 100:463, 1955.
16. Dean, R. E., Isbell, N. P., and Woodard, D. E.: Cervical carcinoma in situ in pregnancy, Obst. & Gynec. 20:633, 1962.
17. Dubner, M. S., Rosati, V., and Duckman, S.: The positive Papanicolaou smear in pregnancy, Am. J. Obst. & Gynec. 88:17, 1964.
18. Erickson, C. C., et al.: Population screening for uterine cancer by vaginal cytology, J.A.M.A. 162:167, 1956.
19. Ferguson, J. H.: Positive cancer smears in teenage girls, J.A.M.A. 178:365, 1961.

20. Graham, J. B.: Patient types in gynecologic cancer, Obst. & Gynec. 23:176, 1964.
21. Graham, S., Levin, M., and Lilienfeld, A. M.: The socioeconomic distribution of cancer of various sites in Buffalo, N.Y., 1948–1952, Cancer 13:180, 1960.
22. Handy, V. H., and Wieben, E.: Detection of cancer of the cervix: a public health approach, Obst. & Gynec. 25:348, 1965.
23. Hecht, E. L., and Oppenheim, A.: The cytology of endometrial cancer, Surg. Gynec. & Obst. 122:1, 1966.
24. Helwig, F. C.: Changing ratio of cervical to corpus carcinoma, Am. J. Obst. & Gynec. 81:277, 1961.
25. Hepler, T. K., Dockerty, M. B., and Randall, L. M.: Primary adenocarcinoma of the cervix, Am. J. Obst. & Gynec. 63:800, 1952.
26. Hertig, A. T., and Younge, P. A.: Debate: what is cancer in situ of cervix? Is it preinvasive form of true carcinoma? Am. J. Obst. & Gynec. 64:807, 1952, discussion, pp. 825–832.
27. Isbell, N. P., and Grover, E.: The vaginal smear in pregnant and nonpregnant women, Acta cytol. 10:87, 1966.
28. Jenny, J. W., and Wacek, A.: The cytological picture versus the histological grade of differentiation of the carcinoma in situ, Acta cytol. 6:208, 1962.
29. Johnson, L. D., and Hertig, A. T.: Carcinoma in situ of the uterine cervix with special reference to the pregnant patient, J. Iowa M. Soc. 48:283, 1958.
30. Jones, E. G., et al.: Carcinoma of the cervix uteri during pregnancy, Am. J. Obst. & Gynec. 89:285, 1964.
31. Kaiser, R. F., et al.: Initial effect of community-wide cytologic screening on clinical stage of cervical cancer detected in an entire community. Results of Memphis-Shelby County, Tennessee, study, J. Nat. Cancer Inst. 25:863, 1960.
32. Kaufman, R. H., Spunt, H. J., and Carrig, S.: Cervicovaginal cytology in the teenage patient, Acta cytol. 9:314, 1965.
33. Kay, S.: Results of the routine cervical cytologic smear in the obstetric patient, Surg. Gynec. & Obst. 114:83, 1962.
34. Koss, L. G., and Durfee, G. R.: Cytologic diagnosis of endometrial carcinoma, result of ten years of experience, Acta cytol. 6:519, 1962.
35. Ludin, F. E., and Erickson, C. C.: Prevalence of intraepithelial carcinoma of the cervix in the early years of marriage, J. Nat. Cancer Inst. 35:581, 1965.
36. Marshall, C. E.: Effect of cytologic screening on the incidence of invasive carcinoma of the cervix in a semiclosed community, Cancer 18:153, 1965.
37. Meyer, P. C.: Diagnosis of preinvasive carcinoma of the uterine cervix, J. Clin. Path. 18:414, 1965.
38. Osband, R., and Jones, W. N.: Carcinoma in situ in pregnancy, Am. J. Obst. & Gynec. 83:599, 1962.
39. Papanicolaou, G. N., and Traut, H. F.: *Diagnosis of Uterine Cancer by the Vaginal Smear* (New York: The Commonwealth Fund, 1943).
40. Reagan, J. W.: Dysplasia of the Uterine Cervix, in Gray, L. A. (ed.): *Dysplasia, Carcinoma In Situ and Micro-Invasive Carcinoma of the Cervix Uteri* (Springfield, Ill.: Charles C Thomas, Publisher, 1964), p. 294.
41. Reagan, J. W., Hicks, D. J., and Scott, R. B.: Atypical hyperplasia of the uterine cervix, Cancer 8:42, 1955.
42. Reagan, J. W., and Ng, A. B. P.: *The Cells of Uterine Adenocarcinoma* (Baltimore: Williams and Wilkins Company, 1965).
43. Reagan, J. W., et al.: Dysplasia of the uterine cervix during pregnancy: an analytical study of the cells, Acta cytol. 5:17, 1961.
44. Richart, R. M.: Cervical neoplasia in pregnancy, Am. J. Obst. & Gynec. 87:474, 1963.
45. Roddick, J. W., and Crossen, P. S.: Invasive carcinoma of the cervix complicated by pregnancy, South. M. J. 59:417, 1966.
46. Roddick, J. W., and Tweeddale, D. N.: Carcinoma of the cervix, J. Kentucky M. A. 64: 505, 1966.
47. Rotkin, I. D.: Relation of adolescent coitus to cervical cancer risk, J.A.M.A. 179:486, 1962.
48. Sedlis, A.: Cytology screening of prenatal patients in a municipal hospital, Acta cytol. 7:224, 1963.
49. Slate, T. A.: The prevalence and significance of the class II smear in the routine screening for detection of carcinoma of the cervix, Am. J. Obst. & Gynec. 92:642, 1965.

50. Sprunt, D. H., and Berton, W. M.: The relationship of socioeconomic and racial factors to carcinoma of the cervix as indicated by a mass screening program, Acta Unio inter-nat. contra cancrum 16:1768, 1960.
51. Stevenson, C. S., et al.: Changing picture of cervical carcinoma, J.A.M.A. 179:930, 1962.
52. Stevenson, C. S., et al.: Detection of cancer of the cervix: a public health approach, Obst. & Gynec. 25:348, 1965.
53. Stocks, P.: Cancer of the uterine cervix and social conditions, Brit. J. Cancer 9:487, 1955.
54. Stone, M. L., Weingold, A. B., and Sanford, S.: Cervical carcinoma in pregnancy, Am. J. Obst. & Gynec. 93:479, 1965.
55. Tilden, I. L., and Nishimura, J. K.: Detection of cervical cancer by cytologic screening: period, 1948-1953 and 1958-1963, Pacific Med. & Surg. 74:53, 1966.
56. von Haam, E.: Should all pregnant women be screened for cervical carcinoma? Acta cytol. 3:112, 1959.
57. Wright, L.: Cervical cytology and intra-epithelial cancer of the cervix in pregnancy, J. Obst. & Gynaec. Brit. Commonwealth 68:771, 1961.
58. Yule, R., and Cameron, F. H. D.: Aberdeen experience in the cytological detection of unsuspected carcinoma of the cervix, J. Obst. & Gynaec. Brit. Commonwealth 68:658, 1961.

CHAPTER 3

Collection Methods

General Principles

IN THE LAST ANALYSIS, the key feature of a good cytologic service is the ultimate diagnostic accuracy. Accuracy is dependent on such factors as the site(s) from which a specimen is obtained, who procures the material and under what conditions it is collected (i.e., presence of active menstruation, contaminants, etc.). In general, we believe the closer to the suspected lesion that cellular material is secured, the better the chance for a positive diagnosis. For example, when cervicovaginal smears are taken, diagnostic accuracy is excellent for cervical lesions but is progressively worse for genital lesions proximal to that area (i.e., endometrium, fallopian tube and ovary).[24] Similarly, it has been well established that pulmonary cytodiagnosis is not nearly as accurate as it is for the female genital tract, in great part a reflection of the distance neoplastic cells are from the collection point in the former. It must also be kept in mind that the morphologic appearance of cellular elements is influenced by the proximity of collection. For example, cells that are scraped directly from a neoplasm more closely simulate the parent tumor, whereas those that travel distances, i.e., from the endometrium into the vagina, are altered by the surrounding fluid medium and tend to assume a more spherical shape.[24]

Experience dictates that the more experienced the operator, the greater is the likelihood of receiving material from areas most likely to harbor neoplasia. For example, the physician with special knowledge and interest in pathology of the female genital tract will perform the necessary visual and bimanual examination, be cognizant of local and general conditions that may influence accurate cytodiagnosis (and so note them) and take smears from areas expected to yield optimal results. Some institutions, during the course of mass screening programs, have successfully used nurses or technicians with special training to collect cervicovaginal cytology. Self-collection methods (irrigation, tampon) are a definite compromise; the best that can be said for them is that they are better than no examination at all.[1, 26]

Certain prerequisites should be adhered to if diagnostic accuracy is to be expected. For example, material for vaginal cytologic study is preferably collected from a patient who has not douched for at least 24 hours. Evaluation of cellular material from a woman who is actively menstruating is difficult. Neoplastic cells may be markedly diluted by the menstrual flow as blood in the vagina may obscure a lesion that should be biopsied and, lastly, the presence of blood makes cytologic study difficult in that it creates staining artifacts, primarily more intense hematoxylinophilia. It is best to obtain material under direct visualization following the insertion of a clean speculum moistened with lukewarm water. The use of lubricant is to be strongly condemned as it seriously interferes with proper cell evaluation.

The specimen may be collected by means of spatulas, ordinary wooden variety or specially manufactured (Ayre), from the posterior vaginal fornix and cervix. A cotton-tipped applicator or aspirating pipette may be used to obtain a vaginal or endocervical specimen. Shute[32] has devised a single instrument allowing for collection of material from the endocervix and portio vaginalis by direct abrasion plus the uterine pool by suction at the internal os. If the endometrial cavity is to be aspirated, one may introduce a sterile blunt metal cannula devised by Novak, utilize a polyethylene catheter, insert a rotating brush[2] or irrigate with a small amount (1–2 ml) of sterile saline.[36]

The collected material is usually smeared onto 1×3″ glass slides. It is recommended that a single clean swipe be made to cover ⅔ to ¾ of the slide. Some prefer to make a U-shaped motion down one side of the slide and up the other. We do not advocate a rotary smearing technique as cells may be damaged or distorted and the slide often is so thick that microscopic examination is difficult. Some express the aspirate on a slide frosted at one end, over which a second similar slide is applied, then compress and draw the two apart. It is important to try to apply cellular material evenly and not too thickly. Any chunks of aspirate that may be on the slide will not stain properly and may interfere with subsequent cover slipping. The slide may be of clear glass, frosted at one end or in its entirety. The completely frosted slide offers no advantage in gynecologic cytology. The clinician will find that identifying data can be conveniently placed on the unsmeared section of the frosted slide with an ordinary lead pencil, which should be done before the smear is taken. Identifying data is ordinarily affixed to clear glass slides after arrival at the laboratory, using a diamond-point marking pencil or India ink. Material from multiple sites also may be applied to a single slide, the so-called combined smear, on separately labeled slides[12] or on a single slide divided into three separate areas.[38] The single combined smear has the disadvantage that it may not be as easy for the cytologist to determine the origin of neoplastic elements, thus reducing the efficiency of subsequent examination and diagnosis. The multiple, separately labeled slides have the evident advantage of more precise tumor localization, but have the disadvantage in that multiple smears are time consuming for already busy cytotechnologists. The single slide divided into three separate areas, vaginal, cervical, and endocervical, the so-called "VCE" slide,[38] has certain obvious advantages. It is less time consuming for the technician, the diagnostic accuracy is high, there is a saving on material, filing space, staining material, and processing time. Disadvantages of the "VCE" method are relatively insignificant and are related primarily to experience necessary to avoid drying of smeared material before all three specimens are obtained.

It is evident that if specially prepared material is obtained from endometrial aspiration, a Schiller negative area, fractionated vaginal cytology, etc., that those slides should be marked accordingly. The technique of acquiring a specimen for hormonocytologic study from the lateral vaginal wall is noted on page 17.

Once the smear is taken, it is absolutely necessary that it be fixed immediately, preferably by immersion of the slide into a fixative fluid, ordinarily half 95% ethanol and half ethyl ether (USP), or merely 95% ethanol. It is also a must that an appropriately filled-in laboratory slip accompany each cytology specimen.

Who Should Take the Cytologic Specimen?

To the practicing physician, the answer to the above question is obvious: the physician himself.[37] After all, he is the only individual qualified by training and background to interpret visible lesions, take routine cytologic smears, and perform a bimanual pelvic examination – all as part of a complete physical examination. The question arises concerning the appropriate circumstances in which a medical student, nurse, technician or the patient may obtain the specimen. In large-scale screening programs, it may be virtually impossible to provide the optimum physician service. Thus, the maxim that any cytologic examination is better than none may be acceptable in the face of inherent drawbacks dictated by economic factors. Obviously, even in such mass surveys, complaints referable to the female genital system must be carefully investigated by a physician, utilizing cytology as an integral part of the study. We do not advocate that a layman be entrusted with patient care, but wish to indicate that, in the course of large survey projects, individuals other than physicians may be trained to take a satisfactory smear. Suggested personnel, listed in order of preference, are a physician, medical student, registered nurse, technician and, lastly, the patient herself.

Vaginal Pool, Cervical Scraping, and Endocervical Aspiration Smears — Relative Value in the Detection of Malignancy

Four modalities, the vaginal pool aspiration, endocervical swab, cervical scraping and endometrial aspiration, are most commonly used to establish a cytodiagnosis from the female genital tract. We will also consider irrigation smears, the tampon method, as well as the detection of ovarian and miscellaneous neoplasms. The relative value of each, especially related to the problem of false negative smears, in the detection of malignancy will be discussed in the next section. In general, false positive rates for vaginal cytology are minimal in a well-run laboratory.[34] Indeed, a few false positives are more desirable than false negatives.

SQUAMOUS NEOPLASIA

FORNIX SMEARS OR VAGINAL POOL SPECIMEN. — Wied[36] assessed the total number of dyskaryotic and abnormal cells present in vaginal smears (vaginal pool), cervical scrapings, and endocervical smears from cases of clinically evident invasive cervical cancer and dysplasia. He concluded that in clinically invasive cancer the vaginal fornix specimens were much less effective than portio scrapings or endocervical aspiration. In the subclinical early invasive and noninvasive group, the fornix smears were only about 5% as effective as the other two modalities. Similar findings were noted with dysplastic lesions. Fornix smears completely missed 11 out of 50 cases of invasive or cervical carcinoma in situ. Richart[27] also demonstrated a high rate of false negative diagnoses using the vaginal pool specimen. For example, he observed 45% false negatives among 97 cases of which 94 were carcinoma in situ and 3 invasive cervical cancer; there was a 63% false negative rate for dysplasias. His study of collected statistics corroborated the inadequacy of the isolated pool specimen. Also, the vaginal fornix smear used alone is of restricted value for adequate cancer screening,[19] although some believe it to possess at least equal accuracy as other methods in the detection of endometrial cancer.[19, 35]

ENDOCERVICAL SPECIMENS. — Endocervical smears seem most valuable to diagnose early malignant lesions, but with more extensive tumors such smears may contain mostly degenerated cellular material. For those cases of carcinoma in situ originating from a squamocolumnar junction high in the endocervix, such as occurs in older women, an endocervical aspiration may be of inestimable value. Most techniques, but especially the scrape and endocervical aspiration, are more effective to diagnose a frankly invasive cervical cancer as well as being valuable in early cases. Because cervical cytology may be negative in around 5% of invasive cancers, the need for careful clinical examination and biopsy, when indicated, is emphasized.

CERVICAL SCRAPE.—It is evident that the location of the lesion dictates accuracy of any one method of sampling. For example, for neoplasms occurring primarily on the portio of the cervix, a direct scrape may be particularly effective, as exemplified by the alpha in situ carcinoma of Old, et al.,[22] or dysplasia. To diagnose dysplasia, samples from a cervical scraping or endocervical mucus are much more reliable than the vaginal pool.[27, 36]

Regarding a routine cytologic schema, we advise simultaneous use of the vaginal pool, cervical scrape and endocervical aspiration whenever possible as they are complementary to one another. If for one reason or another all three cannot be used to collect cells, it seems safest to rely on the external os aspiration and cervical scraping.[27] Table 3-1 is an excellent summary of various procedures used in the cytologic examination of the female reproductive tract.

TABLE 3-1.—SUMMARY OF PROCEDURES FOR CYTOLOGIC EXAMINATION OF FEMALE REPRODUCTIVE TRACT*

SITE OF COLLECTION OF SPECIMEN	PREFERRED INSTRUMENTS FOR PREPARATION OF SPECIMEN	USEFULNESS OF SPECIMENS		
		For Hormonal Evaluation	For Adenocarcinoma of Uterine Corpus	For Screening for Cervical Carcinoma
Lateral vaginal wall	Wooden tongue blade‡ (pipet possible but too cumbersome)	Optimal	Useless	Poor
Posterior fornix	Wooden tongue blade† (pipet possible but too cumbersome; direct speculum also possible)	Good (contamination with cellular debris and mucus)	Fair to poor (sometimes good, however)	Fair to poor (according to localization of lesion)
Ectocervix	Wooden tongue blade (no alternate techniques on ectocervix recommended)	Poor to useless (contamination with regenerative epithelia, endocervical cells, debris and mucus)	Useless to very poor	Very good to optimal (according to localization and extent of lesion)
Endocervix	Premoistened cotton applicator, platinum loop or pipet	Useless	Good	Very good to optimal (according to localization and extent of lesion)
Intrauterine cavity†	Intrauterine brush or aspiration	Useless	Optimal	Useless

*From Wied, G. L.: Techniques for collection and preparation of cytologic specimens, Clin. Obst. & Gynec. 4:1031, 1961.
†Prepared under sterile conditions.
‡Premoistened, if material is scanty.

ADENOCARCINOMA

ENDOMETRIAL. — It has been noted previously that the pick-up rate of unsuspected endometrial adenocarcinoma using routine cytology is discouraging indeed.[16, 24] By the time cytologic studies are instituted, the patient ordinarily will be symptomatic and will require a curettage. At that time, one may resort to endometrial aspiration and expect a high degree of accuracy.[12, 13, 15, 34] Of routine methods, i.e., vaginal pool, cervical scrape, and endocervical aspiration, none seem particularly effective, although each has had proponents. Such examinations may result in a mixture of cells from many areas, adding a dilution factor to an already difficult diagnostic problem; the presence of endocervical cells may be especially confusing.[16, 25, 26, 34, 35] Herovici[14] feels that the combination of the aforementioned three methods are more effective in the cytodiagnosis of endometrial adenocarcinoma than any combination or individual technique. Jameson[15] has evaluated the rotating brush, endometrial lavage and aspiration techniques to obtain endometrial cytology, finding the latter two more effective than the former. The endometrial brush technique[18] and Shute[32] aspirator gather cells from the uterine cavity by means of abrasion and aspiration, respectively.

CERVICAL. — The location of early cervical adenocarcinoma is from the surface and glandular epithelium of the cervical canal. In such instances, endocervical aspiration or swab techniques especially may be valuable to detect malignant cells. When a glandular cervical neoplasm has become large and ulcerative, malignant tumor cells may be collected with great facility by either cervical scrapings, endocervical swab or aspiration techniques. Samples obtained by forcible dislodging of cells have been demonstrated to contain more cancer cells than those methods depending on spontaneous exfoliation.[24] Adenocarcinomas of mesonephric origin will ordinarily not exfoliate early due to their subepithelial origin. When they are more advanced, they may be detected as noted for usual cervical adenocarcinomas.

The Irrigation Smear

In 1962, the irrigation smear was introduced into the cytologic armamentarium.[7] It utilizes a disposable plastic pipette containing a cell preservative. The patient irrigates the upper vagina and then withdraws the solution into the pipette. The material is mailed to the laboratory for processing. Technical points are detailed in the original article.[7] Subsequently, Bredahl, et al.,[5] reported that when the irrigation smear is collected by a physician, it is equally accurate as the cervical scrape, both of these methods being more accurate than the vaginal pool specimen. They indicated, however, that, because of differences in character of directly prepared smears from a scraping and those made from irrigation fluid, it is necessary for the cytologist to gain experience in interpretation of the latter method. Anderson and Gunn[1] studied results of vaginal irrigation performed by the patient, finding a 72% accuracy compared to 97% by the cervical scrape for the diagnosis of carcinoma in situ. With confirmed invasive cancers, the irrigation specimen was 17% less accurate than the cervical scrape. Factors, other than technical, making the irrigation method less than ideal are failure of acceptance by the patients and inability to follow instructions. Others have also indicated that because of false negative rates the irrigation method should be restricted to populations that cannot be reached by more conventional cytologic techniques.[26]

The Tampon Method to Obtain Cytologic Material

The tampon method to obtain the vaginal cytology specimen was introduced in 1954 by Brunschwig in conjunction with Andre Draghi.[6] Made by the Tampax Corp., Palmer, Massachusetts, it is, in essence, like the absorbent intravaginal tampon encased in a cardboard cylinder for use during menstrual flow. However, with the cytodetection tampon of Draghi, the central core of cotton is ensheathed in nonabsorbent nylon. The tampon is inserted into the vagina, usually for 5–30 minutes but sometimes for hours, and, following its removal, the material from the tampon is smeared on two slides. Papanicolaou[23] felt that the tampon method was not as valuable as a set of vaginal and endocervical smears but that it offered advantages over the vaginal pool specimen. By the tampon method, he was able to positively diagnose or alert the physician to the presence of cancer in 97% of proven cases. Unfortunately, the average cytologist can only rarely approach the diagnostic brilliance of Papanicolaou.

Subsequently, Nieburgs[21] modified a Meds menstrual tampon, reporting 100% accuracy in detecting cervical cancer and noted that parallel endocervical smears may have some cases that are negative. Bader, *et al.*,[3] also were impressed with the accuracy of the tampon method. They further noted the quality of smears to be good in 53.7%, fair in 32.3%, and poor in 14%. Of the 2,694 patients studied, the quality of insertion of the device by the patient was good in 59.8%, fair in 10.6%, poor in 5.3% and not noted in 24.3%. Scott, *et al.*,[30] studied the tampon method in the diagnosis of atypical squamous hyperplasia, cervical carcinoma (in situ and invasive), and endometrial adenocarcinoma, comparing those findings with results following routine aspiration and scraping of the uterine cervix. They concluded that the tampon method was inferior to the routine collection techniques in the detection of atypical dysplasia and carcinoma in situ lesions, was as satisfactory as routine methods when dealing with invasive cancer and was more effective for cytodiagnosis of endometrial adenocarcinoma. Some[8] have noted the tampon method to be inferior in diagnosis of dysplasia and in situ and invasive cervical cancer.

It should be concluded that, like the irrigation method, the tampon smear is of prime value only in those patients who will not submit to other established cytologic modalities.

Value of Various Techniques to Diagnose Ovarian Malignancy

Ovarian adenocarcinoma may be detected by using any of the techniques mentioned previously. The few reports[11, 28] on the subject primarily have stressed the use of the vaginal pool specimen. The surprising pick-up rate of 23%–30% of known ovarian cancers by some[11] has not been duplicated in our laboratories. Graham, et al.,[9, 10] have reported on the use of the cul-de-sac aspiration as a screening procedure for ovarian cancer detection, one such case discovered among 186 studied. It is obvious that routine screening for ovarian cancer by any method is subject to the prevalence of the disease; that malignancy occurs only in about 12 per 100,000 women, being 1/5 as common as malignancy of the uterus (cervix and corpus).[33]

Various Techniques in the Diagnosis of Miscellaneous Gynecologic Malignancies

The use of a cervical cap,[17] a jet washer[4] and endometrial suction[29] to pick up primary carcinoma of the fallopian tube, and the vaginal pool to detect a primary Bartholin's gland adenocarcinoma, have been reported.[20] Some[31] have indicated a 60% pick-up rate for tubal carcinoma, although the specific method of specimen collection was not noted.

The identification of endometrial sarcomas may be detected by endometrial or endocervical aspiration. Those extending to the cervix may be diagnosed following cervical scrapings. In a case of sarcoma botryoides, we were disappointed by failing to discover malignant cells by direct scraping, undoubtedly a reflection of the predominant submucosal location of such tumors. However, the value of such studies is more of academic interest, as the disease is ordinarily clinically manifest.

The routine use of vaginal smears in the patient who has had a hysterectomy or radiation therapy for carcinoma is strongly recommended. In a number of those cases, we have discovered dysplasia, in situ or early invasive squamous cancer or adenocarcinoma in the vagina because of positive smear studies.

Pelvic masses, inaccessible to diagnosis other than by laparotomy, can be diagnosed by means of needle aspiration. The collected material may be in the form of tissue and should be so processed. However, should the aspirate be of fluid nature, it can be studied as follows: 1) smearing and staining by the Papanicolaou method, 2) a conventional cell block or 3) concentration on various filters as Millipore* or Nuclepore.†

Needle aspiration is contraindicated should there be suspicion that the condition represents an ovarian mass; breeching of an intact capsule could lead to peritoneal implantation of a malignant tumor.

REFERENCES

1. Anderson, W. A. D., and Gunn, S. A.: A critical evaluation of the vaginal irrigation kit as a screening method for the detection of cancer of the cervix, Acta cytol. 10:149, 1966.
2. Ayre, J. E.: Rotating endometrial brush: new technique for the diagnosis of fundal carcinoma, Obst. & Gynec. 5:137, 1955.
3. Bader, G. M., *et al.*: A study of the detection-tampon method as a screening device for uterine cancer, Cancer 10:332, 1957.
4. Bolding, O. T., Williams, J. R., and Jones, W. N.: Primary carcinoma of the fallopian tube with abnormal "jet washings," J. M. A. Alabama 34:57, 1964.
5. Bredahl, E., Koch, F., and Stakemann, G.: Cancer detection by cervical scrapings, vaginal pool smears and irrigation smears. A comparative study, Acta cytol. 9:189, 1965.
6. Brunschwig, A.: A method for mass screening for cytological detection of carcinoma of the cervix uteri, Cancer 7:1182, 1954.
7. Davis, H. J.: The irrigation smear: accuracy in detection of cervical cancer, Acta cytol. 6:459, 1962.
8. Ferguson, J. H., and Matz, M. H.: Material obtained by two techniques: (a) vaginal smears and (b) cervical smears, Acta cytol. 4:246, 1960.
9. Graham, R. M.: Detection of ovarian cancer at an early stage, Obst. & Gynec. 26:151, 1965.
10. Graham, R. M., Bartels, J. D., and Graham, J. B.: Screening for ovarian cancer by cul-de-sac aspiration, Acta cytol. 6:492, 1962.
11. Graham, R. M., and van Niekerk, W. A.: Vaginal cytology in cancer of the ovary, Acta cytol. 6:496, 1962.
12. Hecht, E. L.: The cytologic approach to uterine carcinoma: detection, diagnosis, and therapy, Am. J. Obst. & Gynec. 64:81, 1952.
13. Hecht, E. L., and Oppenheim, A.: The cytology of endometrial cancer, Surg. Gynec. & Obst. 122:1025, 1966.
14. Herovici, C.: Material obtained by three techniques: (a) vaginal smears, (b) cervical smears, (c) endocervical smears, Acta cytol. 4:254, 1960.
15. Jameson, M. H.: A clinical appraisal of techniques for obtaining fresh cells for endometrial cytology, New Zealand M. J. 60:316, 1961.
16. Koss, L. G., and Durfee, G. R.: Cytologic diagnosis of endometrial carcinoma; result of ten years' experience, Acta cytol. 6:519, 1962.
17. MacLean, K. S.: Tubal malignancy. A method for collecting specimens for cytological study, Science 114:181, 1951.
18. MacLean, K. S.: An abrasive endometrial cytologic brush, Am. J. Obst. & Gynec. 69:452, 1955.
19. Miller, E. M., and von Haam, E.: A comparison of the vaginal aspiration and cervical scraping techniques in the screening process for uterine cancer, Acta cytol. 5:214, 1961.
20. Naib, Z. M.: Exfoliative cytology of a primary Bartholin's gland adenocarcinoma, Obst. & Gynec. 22:352, 1963.
21. Nieburgs, H. E.: Detection of cancer in the cervix uteri. Use of a new method of cell collection, Obst. & Gynec. 7:10, 1956.

*Millipore Corporation, Bedford, Mass. 01730

†Irradiation Processing Operation, General Electric Co., Vallecitos Rd., Pleasanton, Calif. 94566

22. Old, J. W., Wielenga, G., and von Haam, E.: Squamous carcinoma in situ of the uterine cervix. I. Classification and histogenesis, Cancer 18:1598, 1965.
23. Papanicolaou, G. N.: Cytological evaluation of smears prepared by the tampon method for the detection of carcinoma of the uterine cervix, Cancer 7:1185, 1954.
24. Reagan, J. W., and Ng, A. B. P.: *The Cells of Uterine Adenocarcinoma* (Baltimore: Williams and Wilkins Company, 1965).
25. Reagan, J. W., and Schmidt, R. T.: Evaluation of cytological technique in recognition of malignant uterine neoplasms, J.A.M.A. 145:82, 1951.
26. Richart, R. M., and Vaillant, H. W.: The irrigation smear, false negative rates in a population with cervical neoplasia, J.A.M.A. 145:82, 1951.
27. Richart, R. M., and Vaillant, H. W.: Influence of cell collection techniques upon cytological diagnosis, Cancer 18:1474, 1956.
28. Rubin, K. K., and Frost, J. K.: The cytologic detection of ovarian cancer, Acta cytol. 7: 191, 1963.
29. Schenck, S. B.: Primary carcinoma of fallopian tubes with positive smears – 5-year cure, Am. J. Obst. & Gynec. 90:556, 1964.
30. Scott, R. B., Brown, A. M., and Reagan, J. W.: Comparative results of the routine Papanicolaou and the Draghi tampon cytologic studies in atypical hyperplasia of the cervix and uterine cancer, Am. J. Obst. & Gynec. 73:349, 1957.
31. Sedlis, A.: Primary carcinoma of the fallopian tube, Obst. & Gynec. Surv. 16:209, 1961.
32. Shute, W. B.: Three-way uterine cell collector for early detection of cancer, Am. J. Obst. & Gynec. 84:1024, 1962.
33. Tweeddale, D. N., and Pederson, B. L.: Serous neoplasms of the ovary, Am. J. M. Sc. 249:701, 1965.
34. von Haam, E.: A comparative study of the accuracy of cancer cell detection by cytological methods, Acta cytol. 6:508, 1962.
35. von Haam, E., and Miller, E. M.: Material obtained by two techniques: (a) vaginal smears and (b) cervical smears, Acta cytol. 4:246, 1960.
36. Wied, G. L.: Importance of the site from which vaginal cytologic smears are taken, Am. J. Clin. Path. 25:742, 1955.
37. Wied, G. L.: Who should take the cytologic specimens? (Editorial), Acta cytol. 9:335, 1965.
38. Wied, G. L., and Bahr, G. F.: Vaginal, cervical and endocervical cytologic smears on a single slide, Obst. & Gynec. 14:362, 1959.

CHAPTER 4

Fixation and Reporting of the Cytosmear

Methods of Fixation

MATERIAL SMEARED on glass slides for cytologic study may be preserved or fixed in a variety of ways before staining. They are:

1. Wet fixation by immersion of the slide into various solutions.
2. Covering the slide with a solution or spray usually composed of synthetic resins or glycols.
3. Air drying with subsequent rehydration.

WET FIXATION BY IMMERSION OF THE SLIDE INTO VARIOUS SOLUTIONS

Immediately and properly fixed material is a prerequisite for optimal cytologic smear evaluation. Papanicolaou's original fixative was a 1:1 solution of 95% ethanol and ethyl ether. It is still widely used in many institutions, having withstood the test of time. It allows for rapid fixation, resulting in cells that show excellent nuclear and cytoplasmic staining characteristics. The highly volatile nature of the ether in the 1:1 fixative makes it difficult to transport. To overcome the disadvantages without sacrifice of reliability, many alternatives in wet fixation have been suggested. These include the use of the following: 95% ethyl alcohol, acetone,[11] 95% ethyl alcohol followed by air drying, 95% isopropyl alcohol, 95% isopropyl alcohol and ether air dried, 70% isopropyl alcohol air dried and cyanuric chloride solution.

For general hospital use, we prefer fixation in either 1:1 95% ethanol-ethyl ether or 95% ethyl alcohol solution for a minimum period of ½ hour (up to days or months, if necessary) prior to staining. Either fixative results in a final stained product that is of maximal quality for cell evaluation. There does not seem to be a valid reason to use other methods as the solutions are not expensive and may be re-used following filtration. Ninety-five per cent isopropyl alcohol may be used,

23

but the final stained product does not show maximal nuclear detail.

For smears that must be mailed because there is no local cytology laboratory, it is usually necessary to air dry, either before or following immersion in a fixative. In general, such methods are of a compromise nature and result in stained smears that show varying degrees of less than optimal nuclear or cytoplasmic detail. The following are methods for fixing smears immediately and then allowing them to dry or protecting them with a covering solution:

1. The 95% ethanol or 1:1 95% ethanol-ether air-dried preparations (those standing in the fixative for at least ½ hour and then air dried). These preparations may show cytoplasmic acidophilia.

2. Those immersed immediately in 95% ethanol, fixed for a minimum of ½ hour, and followed by an overlay of glycerin, with a second slide applied to the face of the smear.[1] When stained, they may demonstrate cell shrinkage and blurred nuclei.

3. The 95% isopropyl alcohol air dried and 70% isopropyl air dried. Such fixation usually results in stained smears of even poorer final quality than the aforementioned.

COVERING THE SLIDE WITH A SOLUTION OR SPRAY

Methods that cover a freshly made smear with a solution include the use of Diaphane,[9]* a synthetic resin, followed by wrapping in wax paper and mailing. Similar techniques utilize polyethylene glycol,[4] Cyto-Spray,* Cyto-Fix† and Spray-Cyte‡ products where the just-made smear either is sprayed or a fixative material is dropped onto it. Details may be obtained from the manufacturers. In general, we have not found the aforementioned to be as satisfactory as the wet fixation methods of ether-alcohol or 95% alcohol alone.

AIR DRYING WITH SUBSEQUENT REHYDRATION

Nieburgs[8] describes a method that allows a just-taken smear to merely air dry, followed by shipment to the laboratory. Before staining, the laboratory rehydrates the slide in a solution consisting of 25% of 0.5 ml polyoxyethylene (20) sorbitan monooleate (Tween 80) in 1,000 ml of distilled water and 75% of a mixture of equal parts of 70% alcohol and ether. Nuclear and cytoplasmic features using the technique are usually well preserved. Complete details can be obtained from his book. Bonime describes a method to rehydrate an air-dried smear with a solution of glycerin and water in equal parts.[3]

A few technical points are germane. Smears that must be air dried

---

*Will Corp., Rochester, N.Y.
†Chemstaat Corp., Inglewood, Calif.
‡Lab-Tek Plastics Co., Westmont, Ill.

after immersion fixation for convenience in mailing will be more satisfactory if[7]:

1. Fixation time is adequate before air drying.
2. The period of time following air drying and subsequent staining is
   as short as possible.
3. The smear is rehydrated before processing.

Smears using glycerin and Diaphane must be rinsed in several
changes of rehydrating solutions before staining to prevent clogging of
stains and wash solutions. In general, an increase in nuclear staining
time is necessary for air-dried preparations. Regardless of fixation technique, it is necessary that the referral laboratory knows how the smear
was fixed in order to evaluate properly artifactual changes.

Methods of Reporting

Papanicolaou devised the following schema for reporting cytologic
findings[6]:

Class I. Absence of atypical or abnormal cells.
   II. Atypical cytology but no evidence of malignancy.
   III. Cytology suggestive of, but not conclusive for, malignancy.
   IV. Cytology strongly suggestive of malignancy.
   V. Cytology conclusive for malignancy.

In the early years of practical exfoliative cytology, the above classifications provided a guideline that was intended primarily to allow uni-
formity in reporting. However, it was soon evident that pathologists
were devising various modifications, or entirely different means of reporting, and those using Papanicolaou's schema did not reflect unanim-
ity of opinion in a given case.[2] Little difficulty is encountered in clinical-
pathologic correlation of those smears that are unquestionably malignant or benign. The greatest area of confusion arises in the smear report of class III.[2, 10, 13, 14] Such a report may subsequently be proven to
represent a gamut of lesions from those that are perfectly benign to
those of unquestionable malignancy. In some series, 15% of those so
reported were shown to have malignancy,[12] while in others class III
smears were subsequently shown to be represented equally between
benign and malignant lesions.[5] In similar fashion, if smears are reported as benign, suspicious or malignant, the problem of the suspicious
smear is comparable to that of class III. Obviously, if a high percentage
of reports are class III, suspicious, inconclusive, doubtful, etc., the clinician is left to clarify the "hidden" meaning of the report.

With the accumulation of greater cytologic proficiency, most cytology
centers have abandoned classifications that do not use nomenclature
paralleling that used in surgical pathology. For example, one may indicate with a high degree of accuracy cytologic diagnoses as either being
consistent with dysplasia, in situ or invasive carcinoma, as well as the

nature of benign atypias. Obviously, because of innumerable intermediate atypical patterns, the meaningful cytology report often is accompanied by descriptive explanations of findings, as it is almost impossible to include all anticipated changes on a given laboratory form. Our institution's report form (Fig. 4-1) contains the following categories: negative, repeat, dysplasia, unsatisfactory and positive. When the smear contains no malignant cells, the corresponding box is marked; benign atypias also are included under that heading, ordinarily with a short description typed in the space offered. The repeat diagnosis is used when there are only a few cells present requiring further explanation or when cellular findings are so unusual that no conclusion can be made; at times, this is our "don't know" category, which we attempt to clarify as soon as possible. Inflammation or other combined factors, such as Trichomonas, severe atrophy or Leptothrix, either obscure or render a reading less than optimal. In such instances, we suggest a repeat smear following therapy, primarily to avoid the possibility of overlooking an underlying malignancy. The positive diagnoses are read as: positive for malignant cells, squamous (in situ or invasive probability so indicated), adenocarcinoma or others. It is apparent that our final standard of accuracy is the histopathologic interpretation, which, unfortunately, is not completely rigid for a given interpreter and much less so among different pathologists. Our clinicians find that such a cytology report can be readily translated to proper patient care. It is not uncommon for us to suggest the desirability of further studies, such as biopsy, in the report.

THE CYTOLOGY SLIPS, IDENTIFYING DATA

Figures 4-1 and 4-2 are from the consultation slip accompanying a cytology specimen at the University of Kentucky. Almost every hospital or cytology laboratory has a different slip, varying only in certain details. Our slip is in quadruplicate: the first page is for the patient's chart; the second, a departmental copy; the third, for the physician; and, the last, a charge slip (Fig. 4-2). The space in the upper right-hand corner of our form is provided for the patient's name, age, room and hospital number, either affixed by an addressograph name plate or carefully written. We do not process specimens without proper identifying data in order to avoid a serious clerical error.

In addition, the specimen has an identifying number that is matched on the slip and fixative bottle (from a detachable tag on the cytopathology form); the patient's name is also written on the frosted end of each slide contained in the fixative solution. If multiple routine or special smears are taken from the patient, corresponding additional identification must appear on the slip and on separate bottles or on the frosted end of the slides.

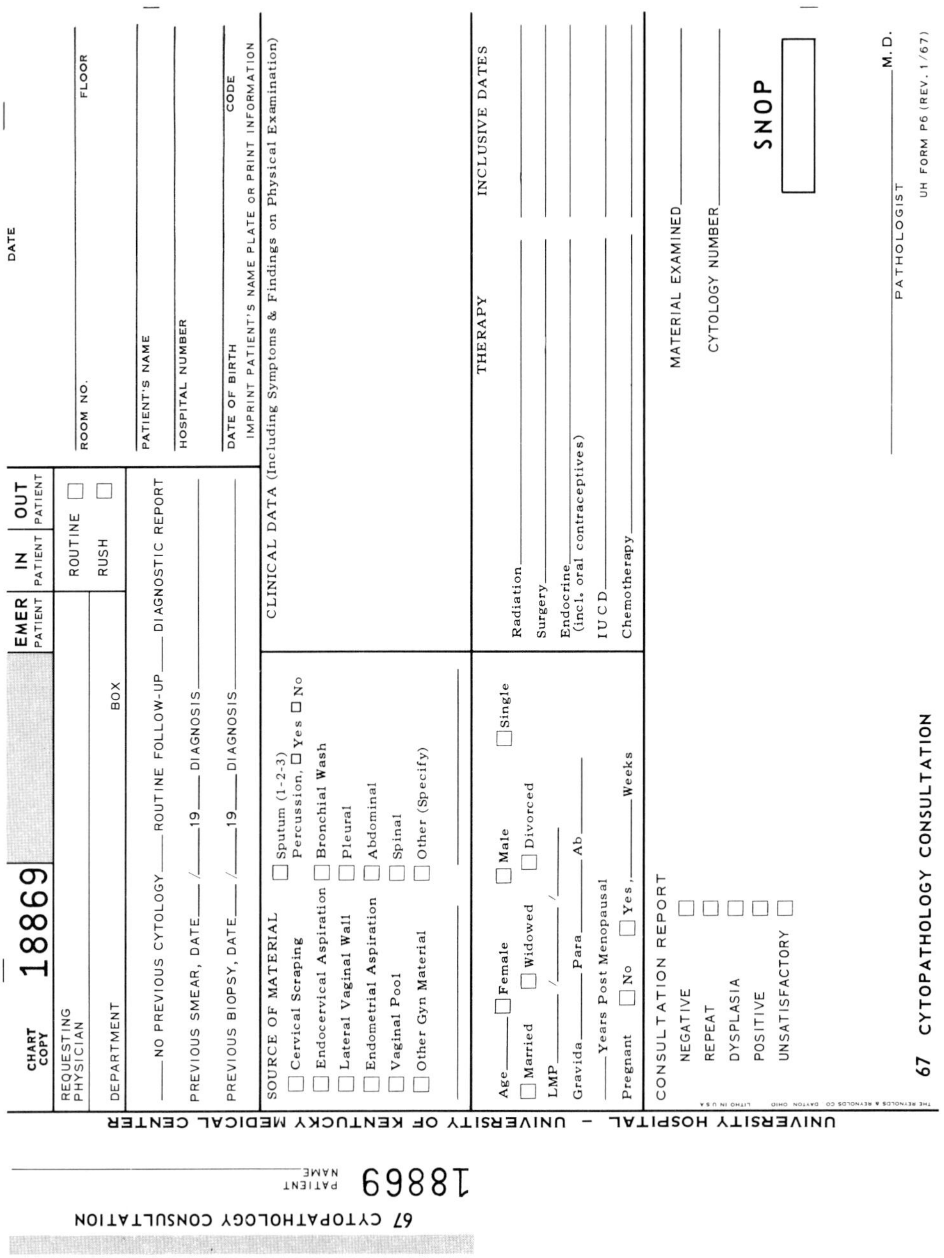

CHART COPY 18869

EMER PATIENT | IN PATIENT | OUT PATIENT

ROUTINE ☐
RUSH ☐

DATE

REQUESTING PHYSICIAN

ROOM NO. _____ FLOOR

DEPARTMENT _____ BOX

PATIENT'S NAME

___ NO PREVIOUS CYTOLOGY ___ ROUTINE FOLLOW-UP ___ DIAGNOSTIC REPORT

HOSPITAL NUMBER

PREVIOUS SMEAR, DATE ___/___ 19___ DIAGNOSIS ___

PREVIOUS BIOPSY, DATE ___/___ 19___ DIAGNOSIS ___

DATE OF BIRTH _____ CODE

IMPRINT PATIENT'S NAME PLATE or PRINT INFORMATION

SOURCE OF MATERIAL
☐ Cervical Scraping
☐ Endocervical Aspiration
☐ Lateral Vaginal Wall
☐ Endometrial Aspiration
☐ Vaginal Pool
☐ Other Gyn Material

☐ Sputum (1-2-3)
Percussion, ☐ Yes ☐ No
☐ Bronchial Wash
☐ Pleural
☐ Abdominal
☐ Spinal
☐ Other (Specify)

CLINICAL DATA (Including Symptoms & Findings on Physical Examination)

Age ___ ☐ Female ☐ Male ☐ Single
☐ Married ☐ Widowed ☐ Divorced
LMP ___/___/___
Gravida ___ Para ___ Ab ___
___ Years Post Menopausal
Pregnant ☐ No ☐ Yes, ___ Weeks

THERAPY

Radiation ___
Surgery ___
Endocrine (incl. oral contraceptives) ___
IUCD ___
Chemotherapy ___

INCLUSIVE DATES

CONSULTATION REPORT
NEGATIVE ☐
REPEAT ☐
DYSPLASIA ☐
POSITIVE ☐
UNSATISFACTORY ☐

MATERIAL EXAMINED ___

CYTOLOGY NUMBER ___

SNOP

PATHOLOGIST ___ M.D.

UH FORM P6 (REV. 1/67)

THE REYNOLDS & REYNOLDS CO. DAYTON, OHIO LITHO IN U.S.A.

67 CYTOPATHOLOGY CONSULTATION

UNIVERSITY HOSPITAL — UNIVERSITY OF KENTUCKY MEDICAL CENTER

PATIENT NAME 18869

67 CYTOPATHOLOGY CONSULTATION

Fig. 4-1.—Pages 1, 2 and 3 of cytopathology form: combined request and report form.

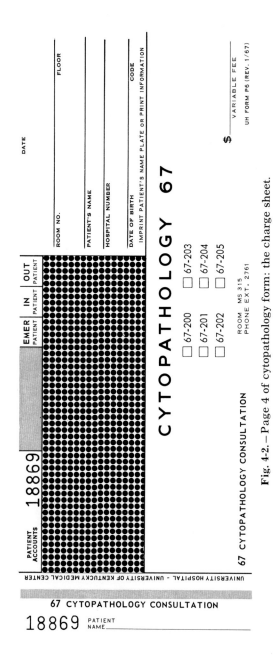

Fig. 4-2.—Page 4 of cytopathology form: the charge sheet.

The section on clinical history should indicate symptomatology referable to the female genital tract. For example, a history of postmenopausal vaginal bleeding usually instigates a search for endometrial carcinoma cells. Knowledge of prior therapy (radiotherapy, cautery, hormone), pregnancy status or biopsy is pertinent, allowing for more intelligent interpretation of cellular changes, some of which may mimic malignancy.

REFERENCES

1. Ayre, J. F., and Dakin, E.: Cervical cytology test in cancer diagnosis: glycerine technique of mailing, Canad. M. A. J. 54:489, 1946.
2. Bangle, R., Jr.: The meaning of classifications in cytologic reporting (Letter to the Editor), Acta cytol. 8:373, 1964.
3. Bonime, R. G.: Air-dried smear for cytologic studies, Obst. & Gynec. 27:783, 1966.
4. Ehrenreich, T., and Kerpe, S.: New, rapid method of obtaining dry, fixed cytological smears, J.A.M.A. 170:1176, 1959.
5. Hall, J. E., and Rosen, I. H.: Significance of the class III cervical smear, Am. J. Obst. & Gynec. 79:709, 1960.
6. Koss, L. G.: *Diagnostic Cytology and Its Histopathologic Bases*, 2d ed. (Philadelphia and Montreal: J. B. Lippincott Company, 1968), pp. 340, 341.
7. Lum, P.: Variations resulting from choice of fixatives, Diagnostic Cytology Seminar, University of California Medical Center, San Francisco, Oct. 10-11, 1964.
8. Nieburgs, H. E.: *Cytologic Technics for Office and Clinic* (New York: Grune & Stratton, Inc., 1956), pp. 207-210.
9. Papanicolaou, G. N., and Bridges, E. L.: Simple method for protecting fresh smears from drying and deteriorating during mailing, J.A.M.A. 164:1330, 1957.
10. Reagan, J. W.: Presidential address, Acta cytol. 9:265, 1965.
11. Sagi, E. S., and Mackenzie, L. L.: Use of acetone as fixative in exfoliative cytological studies, Am. J. Obst. & Gynec. 73:437, 1957.
12. Smith, C. W., and Sealey, R. M.: The clinical significance of class III cervical Papanicolaou smears, Am. Surgeon 28:420, 1962.
13. Wied, G. L.: The meaning of class 3 of the Papanicolaou classification of specimens from the female genital tract (Editorial), Acta cytol. 8:99, 1964.
14. Wied, G. L.: The tenth anniversary of the journal (Editorial), Acta cytol. 10:1, 1966.

CHAPTER 5

The Cell

By Jeptha R. Hostetler, Ph.D.

Department of Anatomy, Ohio State University

Cells are the fundamental morphologic and functional units of the body. Together with their extracellular products, cells make up the tissues of the body. The complex nature of cell structure and function becomes progressively more evident as electron microscopy, cytochemistry, biochemical analysis, experimental manipulation and cytogenetics present new information and concepts.

A generation ago our conception of cell structure was based upon and limited by experimental and descriptive morphologic and histochemical evidence as observed with light microscopic systems (Fig. 5-1).[7] The advent of the electron microscope opened a new era of fine-structural morphology, resulting in the elucidation of cellular structures not previously visible with optical microscopes. By means of the electron microscope, intracellular membranes were seen to dominate the internal structure of the cell (Figs. 5-2, 5-3 and 5-4, B).[7]

Light microscopy is the primary method used to study cells in clinical cytology. The early diagnosis of malignant neoplasms of the female genital tract is made by observing the morphologic and tinctorial characteristics of isolated or grouped cells.[9, 12] These cells are commonly fixed and then stained by the Papanicolaou method. In addition, cells of the female genital tract, whether viable or nonviable, can be studied by phase microscopy. The increased contrast provided by the phase microscope is most useful for observing living cells.

Due to the limitations of optical resolution, structures less than 0.2 micron in diameter, which constitute the bulk of known cellular organelles, are often indistinguishable by light microscopy. Thus, practical cytodiagnosis excludes critical examination of much subcellular structure and depends on careful observation of larger cell structures that show tinctorial differences by conventional staining and microscopy.

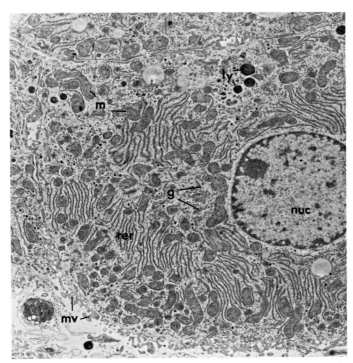

Fig. 5-1.—Low-power magnification of a liver cell from a mouse. Cytoplasmic organelles including lysosomes, *ly*, mitochondria, *m*, Golgi apparatus, *g*, and rough endoplasmic reticulum, *rer*, are shown. This cell has an eccentrically placed nucleus, *nuc*, and shows modifications of the plasma membrane known as microvilli, *mv*. These are seen as small, fingerlike projections radiating from the cell surface. ×17,600. (Courtesy of Dr. Harold Parks, Department of Anatomy, University of Kentucky College of Medicine.)

Characteristics of various normal and abnormal cells of the female genital tract in smears stained by the Papanicolaou method are indicated in specific chapters.

Cellular Constituents

The *nucleus*, which is a constant and essential component of nearly all cells, is the most obvious constituent of the cell when observed by microscopic systems (Figs. 5-1 and 5-4, *A*). The nucleus contains the genetic material, deoxyribonucleic acid (DNA), that determines the specificity of the cell's differentiation and controls its metabolic activities. In cells stained with basic dyes, the interphase nucleus exhibits a basophilia which can be attributed in large measure to the high content of DNA.[8] During mitosis, DNA is localized in the chromosomes, which appear as rodlike or filamentous elements. The interphase nucleus contains irregular clumps which, while not highly constant, tend to be characteristic in texture, quantity and size in any given cell type. These

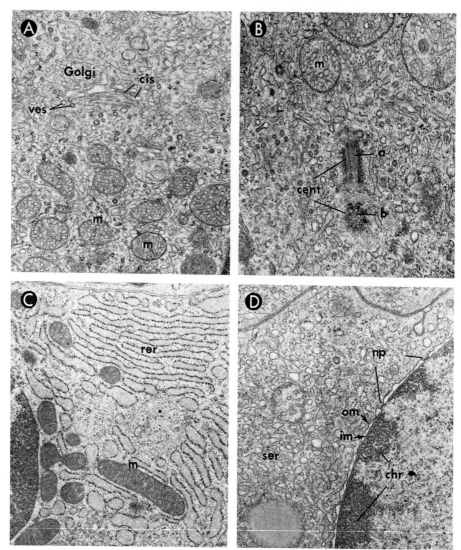

Fig. 5-2. — **A**, the Golgi complex is evident as a composition of flattened sacs called cisternae, *cis*, and rounded vesicles, *ves*. Also shown are mitochondria with tubular cristae. Adrenal cortical cell from a tree shrew. ×31,600. **B**, in cells capable of division, the interphase stage of development usually exhibits two centrioles lying at right angles to each other. This centralized area of the cell is known as the *cytocentrum* or *cell center*. The bottom centriole, *b*, is cut in cross-section and clearly displays triplet units of tubules which form the wall of the cylindrically shaped centriole. The upper centriole, *a*, is cut longitudinally and exhibits parallel alignments of small tubules. Adrenal cortical cell from a tree shrew. ×61,000. **C**, rough (granular) endoplasmic reticulum, *rer*, is seen to good advantage in this figure as membrane-bound cisternae which are studded with ribosomes on the cytoplasmic surfaces. This *rer* is dilated and contains amorphous material. One of several mitochondria is shown at *m*. Plasma cell from a tree shrew. ×21,400. **D**, adrenal cortical cells usually contain an abundance of smooth (agranular) endoplasmic reticulum, *ser*. This tubular, membrane-bound system has extensive anastomoses throughout the cytoplasm. Nuclear pores, *np*, in this cell are spanned by a fine limiting structure. Chromatin, *chr*, is seen in close association with the inner membrane, *im*, which are separated by a space of variable dimension. These two membranes are seen in continuity with each other at the margins of the nuclear pores. Adrenal cortical cell from a tree shrew. ×46,000.

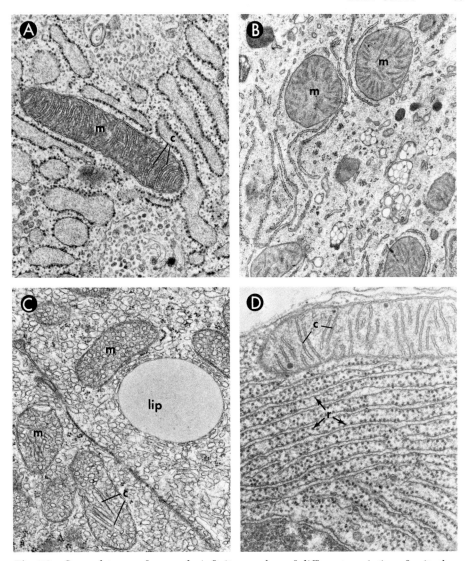

Fig. 5-3. — Several types of a nearly infinite number of different varieties of mitochondria. These mitochondria are located in the cytoplasm. **A,** plasma cell. This sausage-shaped mitochondrion shows outer and inner mitochondrial membranes. In addition, stacked, platelike cristae, c, are seen as reflections of the inner mitochondrial membrane. These sausage-shaped mitochondria have been observed to measure up to four microns in length. ×38,600. **B,** liver cell. Round- to oval-shaped mitochondria, m, in this cell exhibit thin, tubular cristae which are randomly placed in the matrix of the mitochondria. ×19,000. **C,** adrenal cortical cell. Steroid secretory cells often exhibit mitochondria, m, which contain tightly packed tubular cristae, c. These mitochondria vary in shape from small spherical to elongated, rod-shaped forms. A lipid droplet, lip, is encircled by smooth endoplasmic reticulum. ×36,000. **D,** secretory cell from a salivary gland. The cristae in this mitochondrion are similar to those in **B**. Each crista, c, is reflected off the inner mitochondrial membrane even though the plane of section does not permit observation of all the connections. This figure also shows ribosomes, r, as they are associated with the cytoplasmic surface of the membranes, forming the rough endoplasmic reticulum. ×54,000. (**B** and **D**, courtesy of Dr. Harold Parks, Department of Anatomy, University of Kentucky College of Medicine.)

clumps, which are known as *chromatin* (Fig. 5-2, *D*), have an affinity for basic dyes. Chromatin is the representation in the interphase nucleus of deoxyribonucleoprotein (DNP) of portions of the chromosomes.[4] The existence of visible masses of chromatin in the interphase nucleus by light microscopy appears to be due to the persistence of dense coiling along some segments of chromosomes and in lesser degree to the superposition of DNP of several chromosomes. The term

Fig. 5-4. – **A**, plasma cell from a rabbit lymph node exhibits a nucleus that contains a well-defined nucleolus. The nucleolus is composed of two units: the amorphous part, pars amorpha, *pa*, and a network of fine granules, the nucleolonema, *nln*. Closely associated with the nucleolus is the chromatin which also extends out to the inner membrane of the nuclear envelope. ×14,500. **B**, unit membranes can be seen in several different locations in this figure (*arrows*). The plasma membrane, *pm*, cristae membranes in the mitochondrion, *m*, and both the inner and outer membranes of the nuclear envelope, *ne*, exhibit the trilaminar morphology associated with cellular membrane systems. Cell from the parotid gland of a mouse. ×66,000. (**B**, courtesy of Dr. Harold Parks, Department of Anatomy, University of Kentucky College of Medicine.)

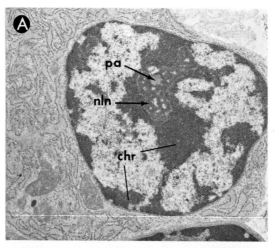

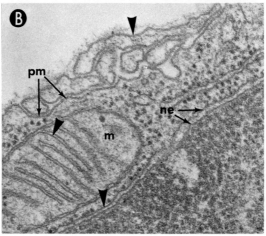

"chromatin" was originally applied to all the basophilic substance of the nucleus, irrespective of its chemical composition. Later, when the Feulgen reaction was developed for the selective coloration of DNA, chromatin came to be used specifically for the DNA-containing, chromosomal substance of the nucleus. Since free DNA does not occur, the term "chromatin" includes whatever protein with which it is combined in its native state. The arrangement of chromatin, sometimes called the chromatin pattern, is valuable in comparing cellular morphology of normal and abnormal cells since the nucleus of each cell type displays a rather characteristic pattern of chromatin. A characteristic mass of chromatin representing the clumped female sex chromosome is evident during interphase. It may lie against the nuclear envelope or in other positions and is termed the *sex chromatin*.[2]

In the living cell, the *nucleolus* is visible as a round refractile body that is usually eccentrically placed in the nucleus and sharply demarcated from the surrounding nucleoplasm (Fig. 5-4, *A*). One or more nucleoli are usually seen in the nucleus of cells capable of division. The nucleolus is rich in ribonucleic acid (RNA), containing about 10% of the cell's quota of this important material.[14] In fixed cells, the nucleolus is irregular in shape and stains intensely with basic dyes. The nucleolus has been identified as an active participant in the metabolic activities of the cell, such as nucleic acid metabolism and protein synthesis. Following silver impregnation of favorable material, it is possible to see with the light microscope that the nucleolus proper is made up of at least two components, an apparently structureless *pars amorpha* and a *nucleolonema*, which is formed by a network of broad strands consisting of tiny granules 150 Å in diameter (Fig. 5-4, *A*). In the interphase nucleus, small spherical Feulgen-positive bodies of variable size and number are found in close association with or at some distance from the nucleolus. These bodies are often referred to as *heterochromatin* or perinucleolar *karyosomes*.

The entire contents of the nucleus is bounded by a double limiting membrane known as the *nuclear envelope* (Fig. 5-4, *A*). At the electron microscopic level, this is seen to possess pores (Fig. 5-2, *D*) which allow for the transfer of a variety of ions and molecules to and from the cytoplasm. In hematology as well as clinical cytology, the profile of the nuclear envelope and the chromatin pattern are carefully considered in evaluating cellular morphology. Malignant cells often exhibit an apparent thickening of the nuclear envelope caused by the accumulation of chromatin material on its inner surface. Even in dysplastic cells seen in cervical smears, the nuclei may be irregular in shape in addition to having a "thickened" envelope.[13]

The *cytoplasmic membrane* is the limiting structure that separates the cell from its environment (Figs. 5-1 and 5-4, *B*). In light microscopy, it usually presents a thin profile in normal cells but tends to appear thickened in some malignant cells. Biochemical analysis combined with high-resolution electron microscopy strongly suggests that the plasma membrane (like the other membrane systems of the cell) is composed of lipids and proteins in varying arrangements.

Specializations of cell surfaces are frequently observed by electron microscopy. The apical portion of the cell may be modified to form small villuslike projections called *microvilli* (Fig. 5-1), which are the structural units of the so-called brush border of light microscopy.[6] Microvilli are frequently present on the apical surface of epithelial cells of the female genital tract. Contact between adjacent cells gives rise to other kinds of specialization. The *desmosomes*, found at certain contact points between adjacent cells, appear as darkly stained bodies in the electron microscope. Fine filaments often radiate from the desmosomes into the cytoplasm. Desmosomes were not recognized prior to electron microscopy, but localized areas of attachment between adjacent cells were seen by early light microscopists. At one time, close attachments between adjacent cells were considered to be intercellular bridges. The electron microscope, however, shows that there is no cytoplasmic continuity between the majority of cells.

Adjacent cells may exhibit interdigitations of their cytoplasmic processes. These interdigitations are evident between a variety of cell types, especially between parenchymal cells of specific organs. In addition to modified relationships in areas of contact between adjacent cells, the bases of certain cells, such as the basal cells of the cervical epithelium, show numerous infoldings of the cell surface that penetrate deeply into the cell. The infoldings divide the basal cytoplasm into elongate, leaflike processes. Mitochondria are found in abundance within these cytoplasmic processes. It is presumed that the membranes covering these processes contain enzymes involved in transport mechanisms and that they are in close relationship to the energy-yielding enzyme systems present in the mitochondria.

The *cytoplasm* is that portion of the cell that is bounded by the plasma membrane and is exclusive of the nucleus and nuclear envelope. The cytoplasm contains structures that are usually classified as organelles. These constituents, including the *Golgi complex* (Figs. 5-1 and 5-2, *A*), *endoplasmic reticulum* and *ribosomes* (Figs. 5-1, 5-2, *C* and 5-3, *A* and *D*), *mitochondria* (Figs. 5-1, 5-2, *A* and *C* and 5-3, *A*, *B* and *C*), *centrioles* (Fig. 5-2, *B*) and *lysosomes* (Fig. 5-1), are the most common residents of the cytoplasm. Other cytoplasmic structures such as fibrils, filaments, microbodies and microtubules are commonly present in the cytoplasm but are not always classified as organelles. The cytoplasm is also the residence of a variety of structures known as inclusions, such as glycogen, fat droplets (Fig. 5-3, *C*), crystals, vacuoles and pigment granules.

Tiny dark granules are frequently observed in the cytoplasm of large, flat, superficial squamous cells from normal cervical smears. These *keratohyalin* granules, which are composed of sulfur-containing protein and an albuminoid substance, are large enough to be routinely observed by light microscopy.

Observation of cytoplasmic staining characteristics is essential for accurate comparison and description of exfoliated cells. The histologic terms *basophilia* and *eosinophilia* (acidophilia) are usually used in reference to the staining characteristics of the cell and are particularly useful in the light microscopic examination of smears from the female genital tract. The term "basophilia" implies the ability of cellular components to stain with basic dyes. In many acid-base staining techniques, such as Wright's stain, basophilia is observed as a range of blue color. In stained preparations, the blue coloration is largely due to the affinity of acidic components of the tissue for basic dyes. As an example, the phosphoric acid component of nucleic acids gives these acids an affinity for basic dyes. One would expect to observe an increase in basophilic staining with an increase in the acidic constituents. Thus, a cell that is active in protein synthesis and has a high content of RNA normally would exhibit marked basophilia. The term "acidophilia," on the other hand, implies the ability of cellular components to be stained with acid dyes such as eosin. "Eosinophilia" is a specific term applied to the incorporation of eosin in sections or smears stained with eosin. The colorations imparted vary from red to orange. Acidophilia is commonly attributed to the presence of basic proteins and hydrolytic enzymes. An increase in these cellular components would result in a corresponding increase in eosinophilia. Augmentation or diminution of cellular acidophilia or basophilia thus becomes an important criterion for recognizing changes in the over-all composition of the constituents of the cell.

Mitochondria (Figs. 5-1, 5-2, *A* and *C* and 5-3, *A*, *B* and *C*), the chief energy producers of the cell, are intracytoplasmic sacs which are associated with enzyme systems and aerobic metabolism. Each mitochondrion is limited by a double (outer and inner) membrane. The inner membrane contributes to the formation of cristae which project into the matrix of the mitochondrion (Figs. 5-3, *A*, *C* and *D* and 5-4, *B*).[11] Mitochondria range in diameter from 0.1 to 2 microns and thus may be observed in living cells with the phase microscope. The energy-generating mechanisms within the mitochondria are now known to reside in the cytochrome chains linked to the Krebs citric-acid cycle. Oxidations occurring on or near the intramitochondrial membranes produce energy which is transferred to adenosine diphosphate (ADP) in the process called oxidative phosphorylation. This results in the storage of energy in the form of adenosine triphosphate (ATP).[6] The mitochondrial membranes are selectively permeable so that mitochondria swell or shrink as a result of chemical or osmotic changes. Thus, mitochondria are sensitive indicators of cell injury. They may swell to be visible by light microscopy.

In ordinary histologic preparations, the *Golgi complex* (Figs. 5-1 and 5-2, *A*) is rarely observed by light microscopy. However, special staining techniques employing silver salts or osmic acid do reveal this important cellular organelle. The Golgi complex, which is usually found in close association with the centrioles (Fig. 5-2, *B*), appears in electron micrographs as a system of small spherical vesicles and stacked cisternae (Fig. 5-2, *A*). The Golgi membranes forming the cisternae may be continuous with the endoplasmic reticulum, and it is occasionally difficult to establish whether a given segment of the cell's internal membrane system is that of the Golgi apparatus or of the endoplasmic reticulum. It has been demonstrated that the Golgi complex plays an important role in the secretory process, serving to store and package the secretory products of the cell. In addition, it appears likely that Golgi membranes are the site of synthesis of glycoprotein.[3, 10]

In living cells, it is possible to discern a pair of minute granules, the *centrioles* (Fig. 5-2, *B*), in the middle of a specially differentiated region of the cytoplasm called the *centrosome* or *cell center*. Under optimal conditions, the centrioles are resolved with the light microscope as a pair of darkly stained, short rods sometimes referred to together as the *diplosome*. Electron micrographs reveal that each centriole is a cylindrical formation whose walls are composed of tubular triplets embedded in a dense matrix. The centrioles are self-replicating organelles. During early mitosis, they reproduce and migrate to the opposite poles of the symmetrical mitotic spindle. Each new daughter cell thus receives two centrioles. In cells that are multiplying at an abnormally increased rate, such as malignant cells, unsymmetrical mitotic division may be recognized.

The *endoplasmic reticulum* (Figs. 5-1, 5-2, *C* and 5-3, *A* and *D*), which was discovered with the electron microscope, consists of a system of variously shaped, membrane-bounded cavities that extend throughout the cytoplasm. This membrane system is observed on electron micrographs as a system of tubules and cisternae (cisternae are flattened sacs or vesicles). Two morphologic categories of endoplasmic reticulum are now being distinguished: the *granular* or *rough-surfaced* form and the *agranular* or *smooth-surfaced* type.

The cytoplasmic surfaces of the membranes making up the granular endoplasmic reticulum are studded with closely adherent small granules called *ribosomes* (Fig. 5-3, *D*). These units are rich in ribonucleoprotein and, when present in relatively high concentration, produce cytoplasmic basophilia in histologic preparations. Thus, granular endoplasmic reticulum corresponds to the deeply basophilic *ergastoplasm* of classic light microscopy. One would expect a cell to exhibit cytoplasmic basophilia when there is an abundance of ribosomes or an extensive network of granular endoplasmic reticulum. Occasionally, ribosomes are observed in clusters and in this morphologic arrangement are known as *polyribosomes*.

Granular endoplasmic reticulum has been shown to be an active participant in the synthesis of proteins for export from the cell. Messenger RNA, which leaves the nucleus, becomes attached to the ribosomes. The sequence of bases in the messenger RNA determines the amino-acid sequence of the protein to be synthesized. Present evidence indicates that protein-rich secretory products first appear in the intracisternal spaces of the granular endoplasmic reticulum and are then transported to the Golgi complex for packaging and subsequent storage as secretion granules. The membranes of the rough-surfaced endoplasmic reticulum have been shown in some cells to be directly continuous with the outer membrane of the nuclear envelope.

The agranular endoplasmic reticulum forms an anastomosing network of tubules. This tubular system is ordinarily not seen to be in direct continuity with the nuclear envelope. Agranular endoplasmic reticulum is probably in intermittent continuity with the Golgi complex and is believed to transport secretory products to the Golgi complex for further processing. Agranular endoplasmic reticulum is found in a wide variety of cells but is especially characteristic of steroid-secreting cells, such as those of the adrenal cortex (Fig. 5-3, B and C), the corpus luteum and the testis. Cells that contain very few ribosomes and large amounts of smooth-surfaced endoplasmic reticulum do not normally exhibit basophilia.

Lysosomes (Fig. 5-1) are present in the cytoplasm of many cell types as electron-dense, membrane-bound spherical units. These small organelles act as the digestive system of the living cell. Lysosomes contain a variety of hydrolytic enzymes, the most common and abundant being acid phosphatase. These enzymes are capable of acting upon ingested substances and, if released into the cytoplasm, can digest the cell itself. In this respect, the term "suicide bags" is sometimes applied to lysosomes. Lysosomes are especially abundant in granular leukocytes and are frequently seen in macrophages, both cell types being capable of performing digestive tasks. *Autophagic vacuoles* are formed by lysosomes uniting with ingested material to break down these substances into usable forms. In other instances, lysosomes may form autophagic vacuoles by engulfing used or damaged organelles of the cell cytoplasm.[5]

Cells of the living body may become damaged by noxious agents or pathologic processes. The damage may be severe enough to result in death of the cells in localized areas. Death of cells and tissues, i.e., *necrosis*, is recognized morphologically by the progressive destruction of cell nuclei and by changes of cytoplasmic eosinophilia. Nuclear shrinkage, known as karyopyknosis or simply *pyknosis*, is noticeable as the nucleus becomes smaller in size, more basophilic, and irregular in outline. Nuclear dissolution, known as *karyolysis*, is evidenced by the breakdown of the nuclear membrane and a fading of basophilia, resulting from dispersion of nuclear contents. *Karyorrhexis*, on the other hand, is a fragmentation of the nucleus into small, irregularly shaped fragments that exhibit strong basophilia.[1] One or more of these nuclear disintegration patterns may be coupled with the homogenization of the cytoplasm and distinctly increased eosinophilia as evidence of localized necrosis.

Although recognition of necrotic cells at the light microscope level is mainly founded upon the prominent nuclear changes, ultrastructural alterations may be demonstrated in cytoplasmic organelles (especially mitochondria and endoplasmic reticulum), even before modifications in the nucleus become evident. One of the first structural changes to occur early in the course of cell death is a severe swelling of the mitochondria with dissolution of the cristae and formation of dense particles in the matrix. (Vesiculation, distortion or fragmentation of mitochondrial membranes may also become evident.) Other cytoplasmic signs of necrosis include a breakdown in the continuity of the endoplasmic reticulum, focal cytoplasmic degradation and the formation of autophagic vacuoles.

The electron micrographs included in this chapter were obtained from tissues that were fixed in varying concentrations of glutaraldehyde in appropriate buffers. Tissues were post-fixed in 2%–3% osmium tetroxide and embedded in either Epon 812 or Durcapan. Sections were stained with either uranyl acetate and lead hydroxide or with lead hydroxide alone.

REFERENCES

1. Anderson, W. A. D., and Scotti, T. M.: *Synopsis of Pathology* (St. Louis: C. V. Mosby Company, 1968).
2. Barr, M. L.: Sex chromatin and phenotype in man, Science 130:679, 1959.
3. Beams, H. W., and Kessel, R. G.: The Golgi apparatus: structure and function, Internat. Rev. Cytol. 23:209, 1968.
4. Bloom, W., and Ozarslan, S.: Electron microscopy of ultraviolet-irradiated parts of chromosomes, Proc. Nat. Acad. Sc. 53:1294, 1965.
5. Essner, E., and Novikoff, A. B.: Human hepatocellular pigments and lysosomes, J. Ultrastruct. Res. 3:374, 1960.
6. Fawcett, D. W.: *An Atlas of Fine Structure. The Cell, Its Organelles and Inclusions* (Philadelphia: W. B. Saunders Company, 1966).
7. Freeman, J. A.: What the general pathologist should know about electron microscopy, Bull. Path. 6(7):64, 1965.
8. Hay, E. D., and Revel, J. P.: The fine structure of the DNP component of the nucleus. An electron microscopic study utilizing autoradiography to localize DNA synthesis, J. Cell Biol. 16:29, 1963.
9. Linder, A.: Suggested explanation for accuracy of the Papanicolaou method for cytologic diagnosis. A histochemical study, Am. J. Clin. Path. 29:43, 1958.
10. Neutra, M., and Leblond, C. P.: Synthesis of carbohydrate of mucus in the Golgi com-

plex as shown by electron microscope radioautography of globet cells from rats inject-
ed with glucose – H³, J. Cell Biol. 30:119, 1966.

11. Palade, G.: An electron microscope study of mitochondrial structure, J. Histochem. 1:
188, 1953.
12. Papanicolaou, G. N.: *Atlas of Exfoliative Cytology* (Cambridge: Harvard University
Press, 1954).
13. Shingleton, H. M., Richart, R. M., Wiener, J., and Spiro, D.: Human cervical intraepithelial neoplasia: structure of dysplasia and carcinoma in situ, Cancer Res. 28:695,
1968.
14. Vincent, W. S.: Structure and chemistry of nucleoli, Int. Rev. Cytol. 4:269, 1955.

CHAPTER 6

Other Investigative Techniques Used in the Study of the Cell

THE VALUE OF light microscopy related to visual inspection of smears for the detection and diagnosis of uterine neoplasia is well established. It is unquestionably the most practical and least expensive of all available examination techniques. However, conventional light microscopy allows for only limited insight into subcellular and chemical activities of preneoplastic or frankly malignant cells. In recent years, numerous other techniques, primarily of didactic nature, have been adapted to the study of neoplasia; this section will be devoted to certain of them, particularly those applicable to uterine cancer. The definitive value of some methods is not established; more data accumulation and technique refinement might hold promise for the future. Undoubtedly, some research tools of today will be routine procedures in the future for the earlier, and possibly automated, detection and selection of potential cancer patients. Only principles of certain research techniques will be presented; specific methodology and other details can be found in cited references.

Quantitative Cytochemical Analysis of Premalignant and Malignant Uterine Disorders

Methods used in quantitative cytochemistry were developed by Caspersson. The underlying principle is measurement of the absorption of electromagnetic rays, ranging from x-rays to infra-red rays, in biologic objects. Energy absorption depends on the altering of incoming rays by intracellular chemical substances (chromotophores) so that a color is produced. Should intracellular chemical substances be chromatophore negative, certain dyestuffs may be specifically and stoichiometrically bound to enable identification and quantitation of a particular material. For example, this method can be used to determine the chemical composition of nuclear materials. Deoxyribonucleic acid (DNA), a chromatophore, can be measured photoelectrically in ultraviolet (UV) light at wavelength 260 mu, or after the Feulgen reaction or gallocyanin chrome alum staining, in visible light. The ribonucleic acid (RNA) content can be determined in UV light before and after ribonuclease treatment. Histone content can be determined by staining either with fast green, at pH 8.2, or meta phosphate gallocyanin chrome alum. Most investigations have been directed at measurement of nuclear DNA content. The reader is referred to several excellent references which detail techniques and discuss advantages, disadvantages and limitations of the aforementioned procedures.[24, 28]

Cytogenetic Studies of Premalignant and Malignant Uterine Disorders

As early as 1914 and later in 1927, Boveri and Winge, respectively, suggested that the transformation of normal into malignant cells is the result of an abnormal chromosome content. Recently, improved techniques have provided a means for detailed studies of chromosome number and morphology; as a result, chromosomal changes in human neoplasms have evolved into an important aspect of cancer research. Because such studies are expensive, time consuming and difficult to perform, our knowledge of the relationship of cytogenetics to neoplasia is still incomplete.[20]

Two basic techniques are used to determine the quantity and quality of chromosomes in individual cells. One method examines in vivo cells – the "squash preparation." The other studies chromosomes of cells cultured in vitro for variable periods of time. The squash preparation is advantageous in that cells are obtained directly from tissue, without the influence of exogenous environment. Disadvantages of this method include the following: there is little choice of the layer from which cells are studied (predominantly surface cells), the cell population is sparse and the technical quality of the metaphase spreads are often unsatisfactory. Tissue culture techniques are advantageous because the examined cells are capable of continued reproduction and probably represent the actively growing cells, many cells are available for study and the technical quality of the preparations is good. Disadvantages of in vitro preparations include the difficulty in obtaining "pure" cells for the initial culture; those cells that proliferate in the explant environment are not always truly representative of the in vivo cell population; proliferating cells may be modified during in vitro growth.

The genetic material within each chromosome is composed of DNA, aggregated into genes, which direct cell growth, differentiation and function. However, despite recently accumulated extensive data, the relationship of chromosomal abnormalities to malignant transformation is not always clear cut. The remainder of this section will relate such data to uterine neoplasia.

Ninety-seven to 99% of normal somatic cells have a diploid (46) number of chromosomes, with a consistent karyotype. An almost constant finding is that primary malignant tumors of man contain cells with an abnormal chromosome number and/or chromosome morphology.[14] Insight into the importance of chromosomal abnormalities and neoplastic development can be appreciated when one observes changes in patterns or deviations in chromosomal number with progressive stages of neoplastic development. Cervical neoplasia is ideally suited to such study where changes from dysplasia, to carcinoma in situ and to invasive carcinoma may be followed.

By analyzing squash preparations, several investigators[15, 16, 36, 37] have identified deviations from normal chromosome number or morphology in the aforementioned processes. Dysplasia specimens have generally had cells with a diploid number of chromosomes. However, cases representing carcinoma in situ show a distinct variation from such normally distributed chromosome counts and are characterized by a wide scatter of chromosomal numbers. There is an increase in hyperdiploid cells, most frequently between 75 and greater than 100 chromosomes, plus a second smaller mode around the diploid zone. Invasive carcinoma cells also show chromosome differences when compared with those of normal and dysplastic cells; there is a similar scatter in chromosome number observed in cancer in situ, although there are fewer cells in the hyperdiploid range. The most significant difference in chromosome number between carcinoma in situ and invasive carcinoma is that the latter cells more frequently have chromosome numbers between 40 and 46 and a second smaller peak consisting of cells with greater than 100 chromosomes. A consistent difference between chromosome number in dysplasia, carcinoma in situ and invasive carcinoma of the cervix would assist immeasurably to distinguish cases in which the histologic appearance is borderline and controversial. However, such alterations in chromosome numbers, while valuable in studying a large number of cases, are valueless in a single given instance.

Kirkland[16] was able to correlate the morphology of mitotic figures in histologic specimens with the number of chromosomes identified by cytogenetic study. Utilizing such data, he observed that certain histologic patterns, not satisfying usual criteria for carcinoma in situ, may contain abnormal mitoses in lower levels of the epithelium and thus warrant a diagnosis of no less than carcinoma in situ.

As implied, chromosome culture techniques produce results that contrast with the preceding squash preparation studies.[6, 25, 26] This difference is undoubtedly a reflection of in vitro cell selection. For example, in vitro study of predominant growing cells from preinvasive or microinvasive carcinoma are, with few exceptions, diploid or near diploid.[6] This suggests that cells that replicate in culture either constitute the growing portion of the in vivo lesions, are merely supporting cells or for unknown reasons the in vitro situation is so selective that it does not accurately represent in vivo growth,[6] whereas squash preparations show aneuploidy to be the rule rather than the exception.

Since chromosomes, consisting primarily of DNA, are intimately associated with the process of cell division, it is pertinent to correlate specific measurements of nuclear DNA with the aforementioned cytogenetic findings. Techniques measuring DNA allow for quantitative estimation in portions of or in an entire cell. Direct and quantitative DNA determinations can then be correlated with the specific cell morphology, without architectural distortion. Thus, early detection of abnormal intracellular change may be manifest before they become structurally visible.

The mean DNA content of normal nondividing somatic cells of various human tissues, regardless of sex and race, is remarkably constant.[19] Studies comparing chromosome number and DNA content in the same material have demonstrated a constant and parallel relationship. For example, an increase in the DNA content is noted prior to mitosis and meiosis or in neoplastic processes. In malignant neoplasms the nuclear DNA content is often variable, correlates with the chromosome number and, at times, with the grade of the tumor. That finding is also supported by experimental data.[1, 7, 33] By contrast, in benign tumors the variation of DNA from normal is negligible.[19] An important bonus of DNA determination is that it may be a sensitive index of the replication process in the absence of mitotic figures, since DNA synthesis occurs in the interphase when mitotic figures are scant.

DNA content and chromosomal number correlate closely in carcinoma of the cervix.[1, 4] When the cells from a large, unselected series of untreated cases of invasive cervical squamous cell carcinoma were studied for DNA content, it was found that the tumors fell into two main groups. One was centered in the near-diploid region and the other in the tetraploid region. The two groups could also be correlated with nuclear appearance in related histologic specimens. Those that were tetraploid were found to be associated with tumors composed predominantly of large nuclei, while the near-diploid group had small nuclei. The two patterns showed prognostic correlation whether patients were treated by radiation or surgery. Neoplasms containing a predominance of tetraploid cells, with larger nuclei, showed a significantly better cure rate than those with cells in the near-diploid group. However, such a relationship did not prove true for carcinoma of the corpus uteri; those with near-diploid-type cells had a significantly better survival than those with tetraploid type.

The number of sex chromatin bodies in cells from carcinoma of the cervix also correlates with the degree of aneuploidy, particularly poly-ploidy, and to patient prognosis. Neoplastic cells having more than one sex chromatin body are generally tetraploid and relate to a better prognosis. Those patients with cells lacking sex chromatin bodies and containing near-diploid chromosome numbers have a poorer prognosis; those having cells with a single sex chromatin body, and near diploid in chromosome number, have an even poorer prognosis.

Not only are there quantitative DNA and chromosomal abnormalities in cells from uterine and other neoplasms, but qualitative abnormalities have also been identified. They consist of chromosome rearrangements within various groups of the karyotype, as well as abnormal chromosomes ("markers") with morphologic features that readily distinguish them from normal karyotypes. Marker chromosomes have been identified in certain cases of cervical in situ and invasive carcinomas[2, 3, 5, 9, 10, 31] as well as in an occasional case of dysplasia.[26] These abnormal chromosomes represent structural changes of one or more chromosomes and have been recognized for years in experimental and primary tumors of rodents.[3] Improved techniques have resulted in more frequent identification of abnormal chromosomes. Additionally, certain abnormalities must obviously exist in chromosomes that are not currently recognizable, for example, changes in genes. Future techniques will probably demonstrate such alterations. The accumulated data seems to justify the inference that some tumors have arisen from a single cell in which a chromosome change has occurred in the preinvasive stage. A wide variety of abnormal karyotypes has been described in different tumors of the same histologic type from a given organ.[3]

Those chromosome markers, identified by either squash or culture techniques, have been correlated recently by Brandao and Atkin[10] with changes observable in mitotic figures in tissue sections. For example, 1.3% (up to 3.2%) of all the metaphases, anaphases and telophases from non-neoplastic tissue contains chromosomal protrusions; tumors without marker chromosomes show only 3% (up to 6%) of cells with chromosome protrusions. However, by contrast, tumors containing cells with at least one large abnormal chromosome marker by cytogenetic analysis have been shown to contain chromosomal protrusions in 18.8% (range 10%–23%) of histologic sections. Thus, the presence of chromosome protrusions in greater than 10% of metaphases, anaphases and telophases in histologic sections of malignant tissues suggests the presence of one or more large marker chromosomes.

Fluorescence Microscopy

Fluorescence microscopy is based on a cytochemical technique in which a basic dye (usually acridine orange) combines variously with the two nucleic acids (DNA and RNA) of the cell. A suitable ultraviolet light source reveals variations in fluorescence of such combinations, wherein the DNA in the nucleus is greenish-yellow and RNA in the nucleolus and cytoplasm is red.[21, 32, 38] The theoretic value of this method is based on the fact that cancer cells ordinarily have increased concentrations of nucleic acids. Potential value of the method as a screening technique for the cytologic diagnosis of cancer was suggested in 1952 by Mellors, Glassman and Papanicolaou.[22] Their statistical evidence showed that the fluorescence intensity of nuclei in cancer cells (using another fluorochrome) exceeds the highest values of normal cells. Von Bertalanffy subsequently described and detailed use of the dye acridine orange.[32] Originally, such methods appeared to be rapid, simple, accurate and ideally suited for rapid screening of smears. However, they have not passed critical analysis to substitute for the original Papanicolaou staining technique in routine cytologic work. Currently, fluorescence microscopy is an investigative tool most suited to cytochemical analysis.[17, 21, 41]

Phase and Interference Microscopy

As investigative tools, phase and interference microscopy can be regarded as some of the best techniques at the disposal of the cytologist interested in the study of living material. By such means, the living cells, most of which are essentially transparent to light in the visible range, are capable of being seen. These techniques are based on the fact that a light wave passing through a cell suffers no loss in intensity, but is altered in its phase by an amount that depends on the refractive index and thickness of the substance. These quantitative techniques are not only suited for morphologic determinations of a large number of cells but can be adapted for evaluation of enzyme activity. Because phase and interference microscopy does not change the living cell during the time of observation or measurement, such means are especially suited for the investigation of the structure of living cells. The reader is referred to texts for the details of the theory and application of these techniques.[8, 35, 40] For practical purposes, though, these techniques can be used to prescreen cytologic material for early cancer detection, for normal cell structure evaluation, and for evaluating microbiologic flora. In screening unstained cancer smears, it is possible to determine disturbed nuclear-cytoplasmic ratio, abnormal nuclear outlines, variation in the nuclear size, thickening of nuclear membranes, irregular nuclear contents, and features of nucleoli.[30] Although this can be a useful technique, it still requires new interpretive experience for the cytologist. The unstained, unfixed smears cannot be stored, must be examined as soon as possible and thus cannot be mailed. These procedures must be followed by the usual preparation techniques for further evaluation of those cases selected as abnormal.[30, 39] We feel that these techniques have unquestionable use in investigation of living cells but, for practical reasons, are of little use as a daily diagnostic tool in cancer detection.

Electron Microscopy

In recent years, the electron microscope (EM) has become one of the most revealing research tools in biology. Its application to cancer has yielded much general information about the ultrastructure of neoplastic cells as well as that restricted to specific types of neoplastic cells. At present, this technique does not seem to have practical diagnostic applicability. In a detailed review of the morphology of cancer cells in tissue, Oberling and Bernhard[23] have concluded that there is no single ultrastructural change which is truly specific for the cancer cell. When all the changes are taken together, the ultrastructural pattern is characteristic, but, in essence, reflects that already identifiable with the light microscope. Electron microscopy has also been applied to isolated or exfoliated cells without greater reward than that of the aforementioned tissue studies.[13] Shingleton, *et al.*, have found, but for a difference in degree, the ultrastructural changes in cervical dysplasia and cervical carcinoma in situ are similar.[29]

Vaginal Fluid Enzyme Analysis

Analysis of the distribution and content of various enzymes in vaginal fluid applied to the diagnosis of gynecologic cancer is still in an experimental stage. The enzymes that have been most extensively investigated are ribonuclease (RNA), β-glucuronidase and phosphogluconate dehydrogenase (PGDH).

In the normal cervix, over 90% of the enzyme RNAase is in a non-particle-bound, soluble form. When vaginal washings from patients with non-neoplastic disorders are separated into cellular and supernatant components by centrifugation, the former has a very low RNAase activity, while the latter has a very high activity. By contrast, vaginal fluid samples from patients with invasive cervical cancer demonstrate a fourfold increase in enzyme activity in the usually low cellular component but only a slight difference in supernatant activity. This correlates with the fact that in cervical cancers 25% of this enzyme activity is cell bound.[11, 12]

β-Glucuronidase activity in both the cellular and soluble compartments of vaginal fluid samples from cervical cancer patients is significantly greater than controls, with almost no overlap in values.[11, 18] Similarly, increased PGDH activity is also noted in cancer patients.[11]

As a diagnostic and screening procedure, enzyme analysis is limited, not only because the procedures are complicated, but, furthermore, they do not always delineate cervical dysplasia from carcinoma in situ, or neoplasia from non-neoplastic controls.[11]

REFERENCES

1. Atkin, N. B.: The chromosomal changes in malignancy: an assessment of their possible prognostic significance, Brit. J. Radiol. 37:213, 1964.
2. Atkin, N. B., and Baker, M. C.: Chromosomes in carcinoma of the cervix (Letter to the Editor), Brit. M. J. 1:522, 1965.
3. Atkin, N. B., and Baker, M. C.: Chromosome abnormalities as primary events in human malignant disease: evidence from marker chromosomes, J. Nat. Cancer Inst. 36: 539, 1966.
4. Atkin, N. B., and Richards, B. M.: Clinical significance of ploidy in carcinoma of the cervix: its relation to prognosis, Brit. M. J. 2:1445, 1962.
5. Auersperg, N.: Long term cultivation of hypodiploid human tumor cells, J. Nat. Cancer Inst. 32:135, 1964.
6. Auersperg, N., and Hawryluk, A. P.: Chromosome observations on three epithelial-cell cultures derived from carcinomas of the cervix, J. Nat. Cancer Inst. 28:605, 1962.
7. Bader, S., Taylor, H. C., and Engle, E. T.: Desoxyribonucleic acid (DNA) content of human ovarian tumor in relation to histologic grading, Lab. Invest. 9:443, 1960.
8. Barer, R.: Phase Interference and Polarizing Microscopy, in Mellors, R. C. (ed.): *Analytical Cytology* (2d ed.; New York: McGraw-Hill Book Company, Inc., 1959), Chap. 3.
9. Boddington, M. M., Spriggs, A. I., and Wolfendale, M. R.: Cytogenetic abnormalities in carcinoma in situ and dysplasias of the uterine cervix, J. Nat. Cancer Inst. 28:605, 1962.
10. Brandao, H. J. S., and Atkin, N. B.: Protruding chromosome arms in histological sections of tumors with large marker chromosomes, Brit. J. Cancer 22:184, 1968.
11. Goldberg, D. M., Hart, D. M., and Watts, C.: Distribution of enzymes in human vaginal fluid. Relevance to the diagnosis of cervical cancer, Cancer 21:964, 1968.
12. Goldberg, D. M., and Pitts, J. F.: Enzymes of the human cervix uteri – comparison of nucleases and adenosine deaminase in malignant and nonmalignant tissue samples, Brit. J. Cancer 20:729, 1966.
13. Greider, M. H., and Scarpelli, D. G.: The application of electron microscopy to the study of exfoliated cells, Acta cytol. 8:39, 1964.
14. Hauschka, T. S.: Chromosome patterns in primary neoplasia, Exper. Cell Res. Suppl. 9:86, 1963.
15. Kirkland, J. A.: Chromosomes in uterine cancer (Letter to the Editor), Lancet 1:152, 1966.
16. Kirkland, J. A.: Mitotic and chromosomal abnormalities in carcinoma in situ of the uterine cervix, Acta cytol. 10:80, 1966.
17. Lawhagen, T., Nasiell, M., and Granberg, I.: Acidine orange fluorescence cytology in detection of cervical carcinoma, Acta cytol. 10:194, 1966.
18. Lawson, J. G.: Vaginal Fluid β-glucuronidase in Relation to Cancer of the Cervix, in Wolstenholme, G. E. W., and O'Conner, M. (eds.): *Cancer of the Cervix, Diagnosis of Early Forms*, Ciba Foundation Study Group 3 (Boston: Little, Brown & Company, 1959), pp. 44 – 60.
19. Leuchtenberger, C., Leuchtenberger, R., and Davis, A. M.: Microspectrophotometric study of the desoxyribose nucleic acid (DNA) content of cells of normal and malignant human tissues, Am. J. Path. 30:65, 1954.
20. Levan, A.: Chromosomes in cancer tissue, Ann. New York Acad. Sc. 63:774, 1956.
21. Liu, W.: Fluorescence microscopy in exfoliative cytology, Arch. Path. 71:282, 1961.
22. Mellors, R. C., Glassman, A., and Papanicolaou, G. N.: A microfluorometric method for the detection of cancer cells in smears of exfoliated cells, Cancer 5:458, 1952.
23. Oberling, C., and Bernhard, W.: The Morphology of Cancer Cells, in Brachet, J., and Musky, H. E. (eds.): *The Cell* (New York: Academic Press, Inc., 1961), Vol. V, pp. 405 – 496.
24. Pollister, W., and Ornstein, L.: The Photometric Chemical Analysis of Cells, in Mellors, R. C. (ed.): *Analytical Cytology* (2d ed.; New York: McGraw-Hill Book Company, Inc., 1959), pp. 431 – 518.
25. Richart, R. M., and Corfman, P. A.: Chromosome number and morphology of human preinvasive neoplasm, Science 144:65, 1964.
26. Richart, R. M., and Wilbanks, G. D.: The chromosomes of human intraepithelial neo-

plasia. Report of 14 cases of cervical intraepithelial neoplasms and review, Cancer Res. 26:60, 1966.

27. Sandberg, A. A., and Yarmada, K.: Chromosomes and cancer, Cancer 15:58, 1965.

28. Sandritter, W.: Methods and Results in Quantitative Cytochemistry, in Wied, G. L. (ed.): *Introduction to Quantitative Cytochemistry* (New York: Academic Press, Inc., 1966).

29. Shingleton, H. M., Richart, R. M., Wiener, J., and Spiro, D.: Human cervical intraepithelial neoplasia: fine structure of dysplasia and carcinoma in situ, Cancer Res. 28: 695, 1968.

30. Smolka, H., and Soost, H. J.: Cytological Examinations Using Phase-Contrast Technique, in *An Outline and Atlas of Gynaecological Cytodiagnosis* (2d ed.; Baltimore: Williams & Wilkins Company, 1965).

31. Spriggs, A. I., Boddington, W. M., and Clark, C. M.: Carcinoma in situ of the cervix uteri, some cytogenetic observations, Lancet 1:1383, 1962.

32. Stevenson, J.: The accuracy of fluorescence microscopy for the diagnosis of cancer, Acta cytol. 8:224, 1964.

33. Stich, H. F., Florian, S. F., and Emson, H. E.: The DNA content of tumor cells. I. Polyps and adenocarcinoma of the large intestine of man, J. Nat. Cancer Inst. 24:471, 1960.

34. Tjio, J. H., and Puck, T. T.: The somatic chromosomes of man, Proc. Nat. Acad. Sc. 44:1229, 1958.

35. Tolansky, S.: *Interference Microscopy for the Biologist* (Springfield, Ill.: Charles C Thomas, Publisher, 1968).

36. Wakong-Vaartaja, R., and Hughes, D. T.: Chromosomal anomalies in dysplasia, carcinoma in situ, and carcinoma of cervix uteri, Lancet 2:756, 1965.

37. Wakong-Vaartaja, R., and Kirkland, J. A.: A correlated chromosomal and histologic study of pre-invasive lesions of the cervix, Cancer 18:1101, 1965.

38. Wellmann, K. F., McDermott, M. A., and Gray, E. H.: An evaluation of acridine orange fluorescence microscopy in cytology, Acta cytol. 7:111, 1967.

39. Wied, G. L.: Phase contrast microscopy, an office technique for pre-screening of cytologic vaginal smears, Am. J. Obst. & Gynec. 71:806, 1956.

40. Wied, G. L.: *Introduction to Quantitative Cytochemistry* (New York: Academic Press, Inc., 1966).

41. Wied, G. L., and Manglano, J. I.: A comparative study of the Papanicolaou technique and the acidine-orange fluorescence method, Acta cytol. 6:554, 1962.

CHAPTER 7

Embryogenesis of the Female Reproductive System

By Harold H. Traurig, Ph.D.
Associate Professor of Anatomy University of Kentucky Medical School

Early Development

A PREREQUISITE TO complete understanding of the embryogenesis of the female reproductive system is knowledge of the formation of the three embryonic germ layers that constitute the foundation of the embryo's general body form. Depiction of these early stages is beyond the scope of this text but may be reviewed in basic references on human embryology.[9]

Development of the male and female reproductive systems is intimately related to the appearance, maturation and partial regression of the embryonic urinary organ—the mesonephros. The mesonephros appears following development of the three embryonic germ layers and the general body form during the fourth week of intrauterine life (Fig. 7-1).

The mesonephroi, which include the secretory vesicles and mesonephric ducts (wolffian ducts), develop in the dorsal body wall near the midline as parallel columns of mesoderm called nephrogenic cords. Growing and differentiating in a cranial-caudal direction, the nephrogenic cords and mesonephroi finally reach and grow into the cloaca. The cloaca is a slightly dilated cavity formed by union of the hind gut lumen dorsally and the lumen of the allantois ventrally, and is located at the caudal end of the embryo. During these early stages, the cloacal membrane separates this cavity from the exterior of the body. Later, the mesoderm lying between the hind gut and allantois, the urorectal septum, begins to grow caudally, dividing the endodermal cloaca into a smaller dorsal area, the future rectum and anus, and the larger ventral area, the primitive urogenital sinus. The urorectal septum, through continued caudal growth, eventually fuses with the cloacal membrane

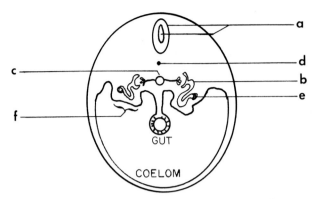

Fig. 7-1.—Diagrammatic representation of a cross-section of a human embryo during the fourth week of development showing the origins of the urogenital system. *a*, neural tube and canal; *b*, mesonephros; *c*, aorta; *d*, notochord; *e*, mesonephric duct; *f*, nephrogenic cord.

at the site of future perineal tubercle (see Fig. 7-6). While the partition of the cloaca progresses, the mesonephric ducts maintain their points of attachment to the caudal portion of the newly formed urogenital sinus. Just cephalad to these points of attachment, hollow evaginations, the ureteric buds, form from the dorsal wall of the mesonephric ducts. They grow dorsally and cranially into the mesoderm of the bilateral nephrogenic cords and induce the formation of the metanephroi or the definitive adult mammalian kidneys. For a short time, the ureteric buds share a common duct opening with the mesonephric ducts into the caudal portion of the urogenital sinus (see Fig. 7-6). Later, expansion of the cranial portion of the urogenital sinus incorporates this duct. Thus, the ureteric buds (ureters) develop new openings directly into the cranial aspect of the urogenital sinus, while the mesonephric ducts (vasa deferentia) retain separate openings into a more caudal aspect of the urogenital sinus. The cranial portion of the urogenital sinus eventually

Fig. 7-2.—Diagrammatic representation of a cross-section of a human embryo during the fifth week of development showing the origins of the urogenital system. *a*, mesonephric duct; *b*, gonad; *c*, paramesonephric (müllerian) duct; *d*, urogenital ridge.

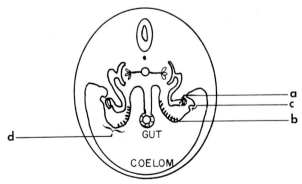

develops into the neck and fundus of the urinary bladder while the caudal portion forms the pelvic urethra. This stage of development is completed by the seventh week of the intrauterine life.

The gonads are derived from bilateral thickenings of the nephrogenic cord mesoderm and overlying coelomic epithelium medial to the mesonephros. As development of the gonads and mesonephroi unfolds contemporaneously, they bulge into the embryonic coelom, forming a urogenital ridge (Fig. 7-2). Later, as the gonads and mesonephroi enlarge, they are suspended from the dorsal body wall into the coelomic cavity by a urogenital mesentery. Following genetic direction, the gonad differentiates either into an ovary or testis during the seventh week and primordial germ cells migrate into the gonad from the gut endoderm via the urogenital mesentery. As the gonads differentiate, new structures, the paramesonephric (müllerian) ducts, develop bilaterally from invaginations of the coelomic epithelium covering the lateral aspects of the urogenital ridges (Figs. 7-2 and 7-3). The paramesonephric ducts sink into the underlying mesoderm and come to lie just lateral and ventral to the mesonephric ducts. The caudal ends of the paramesonephric ducts grow caudally through the mesoderm of the urogenital ridges toward the urogenital sinus. As a result of continuing growth of the embryonic coelom and body, the urogenital ridges, especially the most lateral portion, containing the paramesonephric ducts, rotate medially toward the midline (Figs. 7-3 and 7-4). This eventuates fusion of the caudal portion of the paramesonephric ducts at the level between the hind gut and urogenital sinus, forming a single midline structure, the uterovaginal canal (vaginal cord of some descriptions). The utero-

Fig. 7-3 (left). — Diagrammatic representation of a cross-section of a human embryo during the fifth through sixth weeks of development showing the origins of the urogenital system. *a*, mesonephric duct; *b*, gonad; *c*, paramesonephric (müllerian) duct; *d*, rotation of urogenital ridges.

Fig. 7-4 (right). — Diagrammatic representation of a cross-section of a human embryo during the fifth through sixth weeks of development showing the origins of the urogenital system. *a*, mesonephric duct; *b*, direction of rotation of urogenital ridges; *c*, paramesonephric duct.

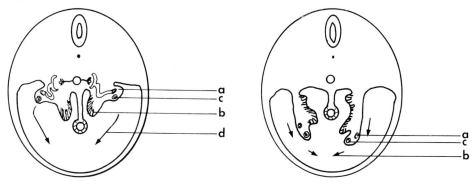

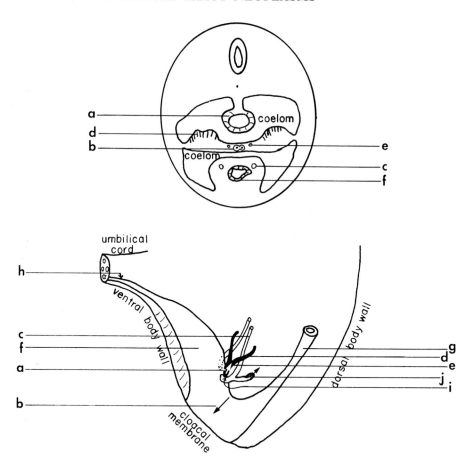

Fig. 7-5 (above).—Diagrammatic representation of a cross-section of a human embryo during the sixth through eighth weeks of development. It shows the fused urogenital ridges. The subsequent fusion of the paired paramesonephric ducts will form the cervix and body of the uterus. *a*, hindgut; *b*, paramesonephric (müllerian) ducts; *c*, umbilical artery; *d*, gonad (ovary); *e*, mesonephric duct; *f*, developing bladder.

Fig. 7-6 (below).—Diagrammatic representation of a parasagittal section of a human embryo during the sixth through eighth weeks of development. *a*, developing cervix. The white arrow at *a* depicts the caudal-cranial direction of the fusion of the paired paramesonephric ducts which will form the cervix and body of the uterus. Their unfused cranial ends will form the uterine tubes; *b*, the arrow depicts the caudal growth of the urorectal septum dividing the cloaca into a dorsal hindgut and a ventral urogenital sinus; *c*, the mesonephric ducts open into the urogenital sinus; *d*, the unfused portion of the paramesonephric duct will form the uterine tube; *e*, the uterovaginal canal, or fused portion of the paramesonephric ducts, will form the cervix and body of the uterus; *f*, developing bladder; *g*, hindgut; *h*, the urachus is continuous with the allantois which extends into the umbilical cord; *i*, the müllerian tubercle invaginates the dorsal wall of the urogenital sinus between the openings of the paired mesonephric ducts; *j*, the uteric bud, a diverticulum of the mesonephric duct, forms the ureter, pelves and collecting ducts of the definitive kidney (metanephros). The arrow depicts the directions of its growth cranially into the mesoderm of the nephrogenic cord (not shown). The uteric bud on the opposite side is not shown.

vaginal canal continues to grow caudalward where it contacts and projects into the dorsal wall of the urogenital sinus, forming a swelling,
the müllerian tubercle (Figs. 7-5 and 7-6). To this point, embryogenesis
in the male and female are indistinguishable. If the embryo is male, the
developing testes begin to secrete androgens, causing cessation of
growth of the paramesonephric ducts. In addition to the secretion of
androgens, it is also believed that the testis of the male fetus secretes a
maturation-inhibiting factor to suppress development of the paramesonephric system. If the embryo is female, the absence of androgens re-
tards further development of the mesonephric ducts. Furthermore, the
absence of androgens favors continued development of the paramesonephric ducts. The most cephalic portions of the paramesonephric
ducts open into the coelomic cavity adjacent to the developing ovaries
and form the ostium of the uterine tubes. Caudally, the corpus uteri,
cervix and vagina form from the fused paramesonephric ducts, müllerian tubercle and portions of the urogenital sinus epithelium (Fig. 7-6).
Certain remnants of the mesonephric ducts persist as the epoophoron,
paroophoron and Gartner's ducts.

Specific Development of the Uterus, Cervix and Vagina

There is general agreement that the corpus uteri, including the endometrium, is derived from the fused portion of the paramesonephric
ducts and the uterine tubes from the cranial unfused portion.[10] However, the origin of the cervix and the vagina is disputed. The more popu-
lar theories will be summarized and selected references annotated to
enable the reader to reach his own conclusions.

The description thus far has carried to the stage where the mesodermal uterovaginal canal (fused paramesonephric or müllerian ducts)
has made contact with the dorsal wall of the endodermal urogenital
sinus to form the müllerian tubercle. This is situated in immediate
proximity to the definitive vulvar area (Fig. 7-6). At this point of contact, the urogenital sinus epithelium changes morphologically and his-
tochemically, forming a vaginal plate which grows cranially replac-
ing the epithelium of the uterovaginal canal (Fig. 7-6). This has been
observed by a number of investigators recently; thus, earlier conclusions[5, 12] that the cervix and vagina are wholly derived from the paramesonephric ducts seem no longer tenable. However, an unsettled
question remains: how far cranially does the vaginal plate endoderm
grow? Koff[6] concluded that the lower one fifth of the vagina originates
from the vaginal plate whereas the rest of the vagina and cervix is derived from the uterovaginal canal (fused paramesonephric ducts).
Mijsberg[8] concluded that the lower one third of the vagina was derived
from the vaginal plate. Vilas,[11] Bulmer[1] and Davies and Kusama[2] suggest that the whole vagina is derived from the vaginal plate endoderm

and that the vaginal plate endoderm may extend a variable distance into the future endocervical canal.

Forsberg's[4] extensive investigations led him to conclude that the vaginal plate forms the epithelium of the entire vagina and the vaginal portion of the cervix up to the squamocolumnar junction. On the basis of similar histochemical properties, he concluded that the vaginal plate was derived from the epithelium of the mesonephric ducts (i.e., mesodermal origin). He further reported that the columnar epithelium of the uterovaginal canal undergoes a transformation to stratified squamous epithelium and then degenerates in the face of the cranially advancing vaginal plate. If this is the case, the postnatal squamocolumnar junction represents a transitional area of unstable epithelium which extends into the endocervical canal and retains its fetal potential for transformation into stratified squamous epithelium. Supporting this thesis is the observation that the squamocolumnar junction is precisely where prosoplasia and the various dysplasias of the cervical epithelium commonly occur. Thus, the reserve cells of the cervical epithelium may be derived from the uterovaginal canal (i.e., paramesonephric duct mesoderm), but with modifications induced by the advancing vaginal plate during fetal life. Their normal tendency to differentiate into true cervical columnar epithelium may be suppressed while their fetal inclination to transform into stratified squamous epithelium is retained. Since these unstable cells lie just cranial to the most cephalad extent of the vaginal plate (adult squamocolumnar junction), they are retained instead of replaced, as was the case more caudally.

Forsberg's attractive theory, however, is not supported by all investigators. Fluhmann[3] concluded that the vaginal plate endoderm replaces the uterovaginal canal mesoderm up to the level of the internal os of the cervix. The cervical epithelium would thus be derived from endodermal cells that have the potential to become either typical cervical columnar epithelium, stratified squamous epithelium or proceed toward some dysplastic epithelial form. This view is consistent with the field theory of multicentric origin of carcinoma which states that since the epithelium of the cervix, vagina and portions of the vulva are all derived from the epithelium of the urogenital sinus, they are all sensitive to the same carcinogenic stimuli.

The view that the vagina (and possibly part or all of the cervix) is derived from an endodermal upgrowth of the urogenital sinus, the vaginal plate, does not explain certain developmental anomalies of the female reproductive system. For example, the anomaly consisting of absence of the caudal portion of the vagina with the presence of a normal cervix and cranial portion of the vagina seems inconsistent with this hypothesis.

REFERENCES

1. Bulmer, D.: The development of the human vagina, J. Anat. 91:490, 1957.
2. Davies, J., and Kusama, H.: Developmental aspects of the human cervix, Ann. New York Acad. Sc. 97:534, 1962.
3. Fluhmann, C. F.: *The Cervix Uteri and Its Diseases* (Philadelphia: W. B. Saunders Company, 1961).
4. Forsberg, J. G.: Origin of vaginal epithelium, Obst. & Gynec. 25:787, 1965.
5. Frazer, J. E.: The terminal part of the Wolffian duct, J. Anat. 69:455, 1935.
6. Koff, A. K.: Development of the human vagina, Contr. Embryol. Carneg. Inst. 24:61, 1933.
7. McKelvey, J. L., and Baxter, J. S.: Abnormal development of the vagina and genitourinary tract, Am. J. Obst. & Gynec. 29:267, 1935.
8. Mijsberg, W. A.: Über die Entwicklung der Vagina des Hymen und des Sinus Urogenitalis beim Menschen, Ztschr. Anat. 74:684, 1924.
9. Patten, B. M.: *Human Embryology* (3d ed.; New York: McGraw-Hill Book Company, Inc., 1968).
10. Song, J.: *The Human Uterus, Morphogenesis and Embryological Basis for Cancer* (Springfield, Ill.: Charles C Thomas, Publisher, 1964).
11. Vilas, E.: Über die Entwicklung der menschlichen Scheide, Ztschr. Anat. 98:262, 1932.
12. von Lippmann, R.: Beitrag zur Entwicklungsgeschichte der menschlichen Vagina und des Hymen, Ztschr. Anat. 110:264, 1939.

CHAPTER 8

The Cervix Uteri: Anatomic and Cytologic Considerations

THE FOLLOWING GROSS, microscopic and cytologic descriptions of the cervix uteri are directed to features that are of prime interest to the cytotechnologist. More detailed anatomic and cytologic studies may be found in numerous treatises.

Gross Description

The cervix is a cylindrical organ constituting the neck of the uterus. Its uppermost limit is the internal os, whereas inferiorly it extends into the upper vagina.[10] It is subdivided into a supravaginal and a vaginal portion by the vaginal attachment (Fig. 8-1). The vaginal portion is visible from the vagina and bares a central opening called the external os. The external os constitutes the opening into a narrow lumen, the endocervical canal, which is continuous with the endometrial cavity above. In the nulliparous female, the external os is small and round, but in the multipara, it commonly assumes a transverse, slit-like opening, often a centimeter or greater in size. The external os is bounded by a shorter anterior lip and a longer posterior lip. In the normal anatomic position, the cervix forms a right angle with the longitudinal vaginal axis, placing both lips of the cervix in contact with the posterior vaginal wall. Thus, the anterior lip lies inferior to the posterior lip. The external os in the classic sense is said to be a junctional area where the squamous epithelium of the vaginal portion meets with columnar epithelium of the endocervical canal. The latter extends upwards to the internal os where there is a fairly abrupt junction with the endometrium. The detailed topography of the endocervical canal demonstrates an imperfectly round tube with numerous oblique folds running in a general superior-inferior direction. The folds branch in an irregular pattern resembling the branching of a tree, so that they are referred to as arbor vitae uteri or, more commonly, plicae palmatae. The deeper portions of the folds are referred to as clefts[5] (Fig. 8-2).

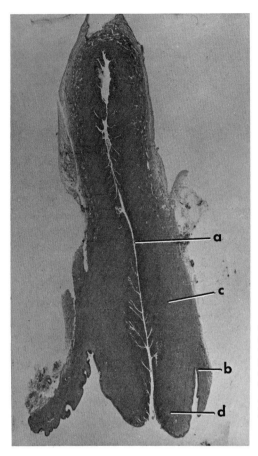

Fig. 8-1. – Uterus from an 18-month-old infant. Notice that the cervix is similar in size to that of the corpus uteri. The area of the internal os is indicated by *a*. The upper portion (fornix) of the vagina is indicated by *b*. Thus, the cervix is subdivided into two areas, the supravaginal, *c*, and vaginal portion, *d*.

There is wide variation in the size of the cervix relative to the upper portion of the uterus or the corpus uteri. In the neonate, the cervix is similar in size to the corpus, whereas in the adult parous female, the cervix is only about 1/3 as large as the corpus. With advanced senility and uterine involution, the cervix may again become about the same size as the corpus. This is explained in part by the lower sensitivity of the cervix, compared to the corpus, to the effects of estrogen withdrawal.

Microscopic Description

Histologically, there are three major tissues that form the cervix uteri. They are the covering stratified squamous mucous epithelium of the vaginal portion, primarily mucus-producing columnar epithelium of the endocervical canal, and the stroma which is mostly composed of fibrous connective tissue. The stroma also contains a few strands of smooth muscle, occasional lymph follicles, blood vessels, lymphatics, nerves, nerve endings, ganglion cells and, not uncommonly, derivatives of the mesonephric (wolffian ducts).

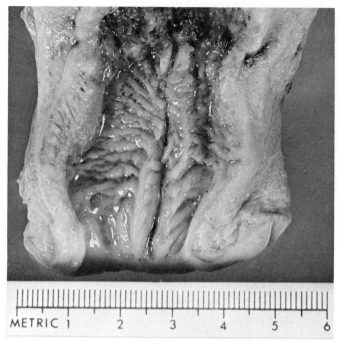

Fig. 8-2. – A normal cervix from a woman in active menstrual life. At the lower portion of the picture, there is a sharply demarcated squamocolumnar junction. The endocervical canal has numerous, mostly oblique, branching folds, the arbor vitae uteri or plicae palmatae.

Squamous Epithelium

Histology. – The squamous epithelium is of greatest interest to the cytologist since the majority of epithelial abnormalities will involve those cells. In order to appreciate the pathologic alterations, a firm knowledge of normal histology is indispensable. Such knowledge can be readily transferred to cytology. The stratified squamous epithelium of the uterine cervix varies from less than 10 to approximately 50 cells in thickness, dependent on the age of the patient or the stage of the menstrual cycle (Fig. 8-3). The epithelium is characteristically thin in prepubertal and postmenopausal females (Fig. 8-3, D and E) and thick during active menstrual life (Fig. 8-3, C). Although normal cyclic variations occur in the epithelium during the course of the menstrual cycle, they are difficult to visualize with histologic techniques. Subepithelial papillae are poorly defined or absent in the cervical epithelium. Five zones or cell layers comprise the epithelial covering.[3, 13] Classically, they are designated from the lowermost position (juxtastromal) to the luminal border: 1) stratum cylindricum (inner basal zone), 2) stratum spinosum profundum (outer basal or parabasal zone), 3) stratum spinosum super-

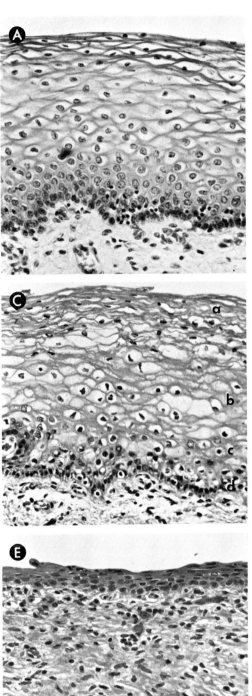

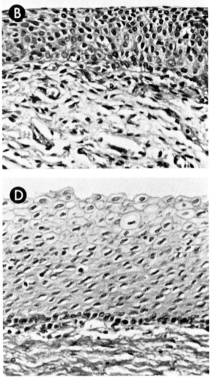

Fig. 8-3. – Cervical squamous epithelium. **A**, eight-day-old infant. The thickened epithelium reflects transplacental transfer of maternal hormones. **B**, eighteen-month-old infant. The low epithelium is a result of a significant deficiency of female hormones, particularly estrogen. Compare with **A**.

C, woman in the active menstrual life period. Cell size increases progressively from the basal to the most superficial zone, whereas nuclear size decreases progressively. **D**, 51-year-old woman who died of metastatic breast cancer. When compared with **C**, it is apparent that the epithelium is lower and that the cells have not matured past the parabasal type. The changes most likely represent estrogen deficiency. **E**, 63-year-old woman. Note that the epithelium is markedly atrophic and that most cells constituting the mucous membrane are of the basal type.

ficiale (intermediate or navicular zone), 4) stratum granulosum (intraepithelial zone or verhornungszone of Dierks) and 5) stratum corneum (cornified or squamous zone) (see Table below).

Cells of the cervical squamous epithelium increase in size from the generally cuboidal one of the stratum cylindricum to the plaque-like, most superficial, cell with a corresponding decrease in nuclear size. Thus, the nuclear/cytoplasmic ratio progressively decreases from the lowermost to the superficial cell. For example, Foraker[6] found that nuclei of the stratum cylindricum were about 32 μ^2 and the superficial layer about 20 μ^2. The area occupied by nuclei of cells of the stratum cylindricum was about 43%, the middle layer about 10% and the superficial layer about 4%. His measurements were made from normal epithelium adjacent to invasive carcinoma, intraepithelial carcinoma and squamous metaplasia. Such histologic findings are readily translated to the field of cytology.

In the normal cervical squamous epithelium, only cells from the stratum cylindricum and stratum spinosum profundum are metabolically active in that they show various degrees of H^3 thymidine uptake, from 2.5% to 10.3%. Such activity is not significantly greater in pregnant females.[11]

CYTOLOGY.—As indicated, the cervical squamous epithelium consists of five distinct layers of cells. Certain layers correspond to cells seen in cytologic preparations and the terminology used follows the majority opinion of the 1958 International Academy of Gynecological Cytology.[7] Nomenclature should be chosen carefully to eliminate terms that are not scientifically correct.[18]

For practical purposes, the cytologist is able to identify cells that originate in three of the epithelial layers with reasonable certainty. They are those of the superficial, intermediate and parabasal types. With experience, cells may be fairly accurately delineated as to the depth from which they originate. It is of great importance to be able to recognize easily normal cellular components during various periods of the menstrual cycle, in the premenarchal and postmenopausal years. Such knowledge facilitates the identification of neoplastic elements. Under

RELATIONSHIP OF HISTOLOGIC AND CYTOLOGIC TERMINOLOGY

HISTOLOGIC TERMINOLOGY	CYTOLOGIC TERMINOLOGY
Stratum cylindricum (inner basal zone)	Germinal cell
Stratum spinosum profundum (outer basal or parabasal zone)	Parabasal cell
Stratum spinosum superficiale (intermediate or navicular zone)	Intermediate cell
Stratum granulosum (intraepithelial zone or verhornungszone of Dierks) Stratum corneum (cornified or squamous zone)	Superficial cell

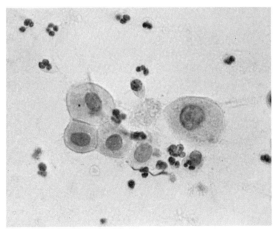

Fig. 8-4.—The two largest cells are of parabasal type, while the small epithelial cells are most likely of basal origin. The tissue counterpart of the latter is indicated by *d* in Figure 8-3, *C*.

ordinary circumstances, basal cells are not exfoliated. Parabasal cells are seen infrequently during active menstrual life but usually form the predominant pattern in early and later life.

The following are brief descriptions of commonly seen benign cells in cervicovaginal material stained by the Papanicolaou method. It will be noted that there is a general increase in size of squamous epithelial cells and a progressive decrease in the nuclear/cytoplasmic ratio from the basal to superficial layers. Nuclei of squamous cells usually are round to oval and vary from vesicular to pyknotic, the former noted in deeper layers and the latter in those cells of the superficial zone.

Basal (germinal cell).—Basal cells are usually oval and quite small, with a large, round or oval nucleus occupying a relatively large area (one third of total cell size). Chromatin granules and nucleoli are commonly observed. The cyanophilic cytoplasm is not as transparent as that of cells from the more superficial area. Such cells are very rarely found in cervicovaginal smears (Fig. 8-4).[7, 13, 19, 20]

Parabasal cell.—Larger than basal cells, parabasal cells vary in morphology from round to oval, depending on whether they originate closer to the basal or the intermediate cell layer. They are characterized by a centrally placed, round or oval vesicular nucleus, often with chromatin granules and chromocenters. The cytoplasm is ordinarily cyanophilic, may show fine vacuoles, and is not as transparent as that of intermediate cells. Intracytoplasmic glycogen may or may not be present.

In menstruating women, parabasal cells comprise 5% or less of the total exfoliated cell population but they are seen commonly during childhood, in the perimenarchal period, following delivery, in the postmenopausal years and in periods of estrogen deficiency (Fig. 8-5).[7, 13, 19, 20]

Intermediate cell.—Intermediate cells are larger than parabasal cells and are characteristically angular or elliptical. The thin, translucent

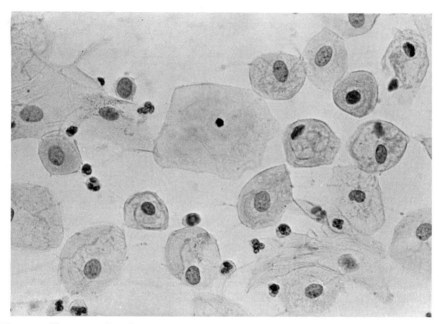

Fig. 8-5. – These parabasal cells are represented in the tissue phase by c in Figure 8-3, C. There is a superficial cell in the center of the field for size comparison. A few scattered polymorphonuclear leukocytes are also present.

Fig. 8-6. – These are intermediate cells, the tissue counterpart being represented by b in Figure 8-3, C. There are scattered Döderlein bacilli.

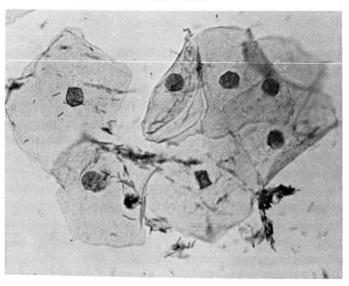

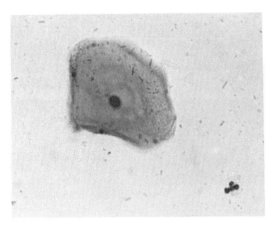

Fig. 8-7. – A superficial squamous epithelial cell. The tissue counterpart is indicated by *a* in Figure 8-3, C. Döderlein bacilli are also present.

cytoplasm is usually blue-green or, at times, eosinophilic, especially in cells about to undergo pyknosis before assuming a superficial cell position. The vesicular nucleus is round to oval and may be slightly eccentric. These cells predominate under the influence of progestogens, cortisone and, at times, androgen, in the second half of the menstrual cycle or pregnancy and, at times, postmenopausally (Fig. 8-6).

A similar but modified cell from the same epithelial layer (stratum spinosum superficiale) predominates during pregnancy: the navicular cell. Characteristically, "naviculars" have larger nuclei in relation to cell size and a thicker cytoplasmic membrane that frequently curls or folds so that the cell resembles a boat.[7, 13, 19, 20]

Superficial cell. – With few exceptions, the largest cells exfoliated from the cervical epithelium are superficial cells. They are characteristically polygonal with squared-off sharp edges, but may be round or oval in shape. In common with the intermediate cell, the cytoplasm is translucent but usually eosinophilic. Rarely, the cytoplasm of mature superficial cells stains blue-green. The most characteristic feature is a pyknotic nucleus, ordinarily less than 6μ in diameter, with dense amorphous chromatin (Fig. 8-7). True nuclear pyknosis is best determined by phase-contrast microscopy. Exfoliation of similar cells with eosinophilic cytoplasm but devoid of a nucleus is usually indicative of leukoplakia, or possibly a contamination of cells from a cutaneous surface.

Superficial cells are in the majority during the first half of the menstrual cycle. They are stimulated by estrogen administration, but may be seen, at times, during postmenopausal years.[7, 13, 19, 20]

COLUMNAR EPITHELIUM

HISTOLOGY. – The endocervical canal is lined by tall columnar mucus-producing cells, usually arranged in single rows, resembling a picket

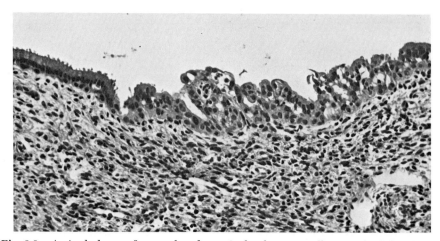

Fig. 8-8.—A single layer of normal endocervical columnar cells is to the left. Although the columnar epithelium of the cervix is composed of cells that are mucus producing, ciliated and intercalated, the former predominate so overwhelmingly that the latter two types are not readily recognized. On the right side, there are several layers of reserve, or prosoplastic, cells under the columnar epithelium, a common finding in cervical biopsies.

fence. The cells are secretory and ciliated but only rarely intercalated — peg or stiftzellen (Fig. 8-8).[12]

The ciliated cells are difficult to see in conventional hematoxylin and eosin preparations since the mucous secretion often obscures the cilia. Ciliated cells are not as commonly or easily observed as they are in the endometrium. Unfortunately, this cell type cannot be easily identified using conventional Papanicolaou fixation and staining techniques. They are better seen in wet saline mounts. Ciliated cells have basally oriented, round-to-oval nuclei with a single, round, prominent nucleolus. Mucous secretion is not present in these cells. Electron microscopy has demonstrated that each cilium consists of nine peripheral and two central tubes continuous with a distinct row of cytoplasmic anchoring granules called basal bodies.[12]

Mucous columnar cells are the predominating cell type in the endocervical canal. The nucleus is generally in the lower half of the cell near the basement membrane. It occupies about 34%–40% of total cell area, has finely dispersed chromatin and a central, single, round, prominent nucleolus. The nucleus may be indented due to the accumulated mucous secretion that fills the cytoplasm (Fig. 8-8). Electron microscopy has shown the mucus to be dispersed in numerous droplets of varying size.[12] Cyclical changes most likely occur in such cells although such changes are difficult to define in the human.[1, 14] Secretion is probably released at the time of ovulation with a consequent reduction in the epithelial thickness. At times one may observe small cytoplasmic protrusions on the cell surface representing active secretion. Secretory cells may become enlarged, forming goblet cells. In the aged, the epithelium is generally lower than in the actively menstruating woman.

Intercalated cells represent compressed secretory cells and are observed uncommonly in histologic sections or cytologic material.[15]

Reserve cells are small and irregular in outline with a centrally located nucleus. They lie on the basement membrane between the taller columnar epithelium. Secretion may be present in their cytoplasm and varies from almost none to abundant. This supports the thesis that they are relatively undifferentiated cells that may differentiate into mucous cells, although transformation of them to squamous epithelium is more certain. Usually less than 1% of the endocervical columnar cells show mitotic figures. They are metabolically active as reflected by H[3] thymidine uptake in up to 6% of cells, especially during pregnancy.[11]

CYTOLOGY.—When exfoliated, columnar cells may appear singly, in strips or in sheets. The constituent elements are predominantly secretory cells but also reflect the other Müllerian cell types, intercalated cells and ciliated cells. It is probable that the columnar cells of the cervix have cyclic variations, reflected clinically by the change in character and amount of mucus during the menstrual cycle, but such changes are difficult to perceive with cytologic or histopathologic techniques. When seen in the smear, cells vary from columnar to polygonal, depending on the perspective from which they are viewed. Indeed, if they are clustered and seen on end, they resemble a honeycomb. The cytoplasm of secretory cells may be granular, vacuolated diffusely or contain a single vacuole. Cytoplasm usually stains cyanophilic but in large cell clusters it may frequently be acidophilic. The nuclear-cytoplasmic

Fig. 8-9.—These are normal endocervical columnar cells. The abundant cytoplasm is colorless or stains a faint cyanophilic color. Intracytoplasmic mucus may appear as a single vacuole or be finely dispersed. The nucleus is round to oval, is situated at one end of the cell and occupies less than half of total cell area. Notice the finely dispersed chromatin; there is usually a single nucleolus.

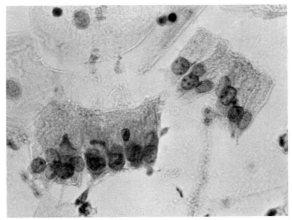

ratio is slightly over 1:2. The round or oval nucleus has finely dispersed chromatin and usually contains a single nucleolus although, at times, several small, regular, acidophilic nucleoli are noted (Fig. 8-9). Nuclear chromatin material may protrude at one end as a small bleb, considered by some to be synchronous with peak estrogen activity.

Nonsecretory cells are similar except that the cytoplasm has a uniform, fine foamy, and slightly basophilic cytoplasm, at times with a few small, scattered, acidophilic granules. However, nonsecretory columnar cells do not contain large cytoplasmic vacuoles. Ciliated cells are broad on their luminal borders, along which a terminal plate may be seen. Numerous fine cilia, several microns long, protrude from this plate parallel to the long axis of the cell. The morphology of these cells can be observed readily in wet preparations and are more commonly observed during postmenopausal years.[13, 15, 19]

SQUAMOCOLUMNAR JUNCTION (TRANSITIONAL ZONE): RESERVE CELLS

HISTOLOGY. – The microscopic location of the squamocolumnar junction is at a distinct variance from the classic textbook example where it is said to meet at the external cervical os.[9] In fact, Kaufmann and Ober encountered the classic location of that junction only once among 853 cervices examined. Their observations also revealed various junctional patterns in that squamous and columnar epithelium may be in direct continuity, squamous epithelium may overgrow cervical glands for a short distance, the lowermost cervical gland may occur in the cervical canal, at the external os or on the vaginal portion of the cervix. The

Fig. 8-10. – Endocervical columnar epithelium is to the left. Reserve cells have proliferated beneath the columnar cells, which are now seen as a single, flattened, superficial layer.

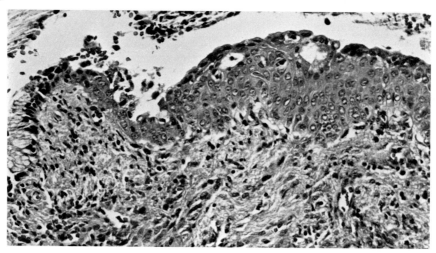

squamous epithelium can be situated a fair distance out on the vaginal portion of the cervix or extend into the endocervical canal.

Certain predictable locations of the squamocolumnar junction are noted in different age periods.[9] In the neonate, that junction is frequently on the vaginal portion of the cervix. In a short period of time, it is located near the external os of the endocervical canal. Upon reaching childbearing age, mucous glands and the squamocolumnar junction are usually seen on the vaginal portion, although the junction may occur in the endocervical canal. With senility, mucous glands commonly appear at the external os or even higher, while the squamocolumnar junction is commonly in the endocervical canal. In one third of the cases, the two cervical lips will show a different behavior of the epithelia.

A sharply demarcated squamocolumnar junction is not common due to proliferation of "reserve" cells creating a transitional area between pure squamous and columnar epithelium (Fig. 8-10). The transitional zone may vary from 1 to 10 millimeters in length. This process in the

Fig. 8-11. – This is a sharply demarcated squamocolumnar junction from a woman with normal cervix. In many patients, reserve cells form a transitional area between columnar and squamous epithelium.

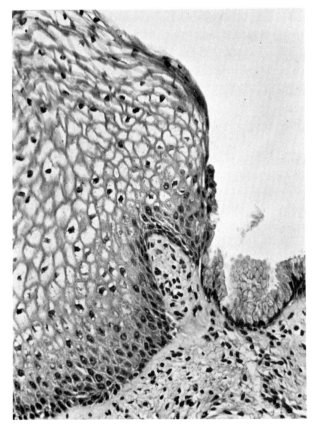

squamocolumnar junction is possibly related to cell breakdown and repair and has been termed prosoplasia.[4] Graham[8] studied 93 fetal and child cervices and recognized two types of squamocolumnar junction, transitional and abrupt. The character of the epithelial junction is closely related to age. This suggests a positive relationship between estrogen stimulation and abrupt junctions since 82% of junctions associated with estrogen-stimulated epithelium were abrupt, whereas only 21% of junctions associated with estrogen deficiency were abrupt (Fig. 8-11). That epithelium of the transitional type squamocolumnar junction is often referred to as "reserve cell hyperplasia" or prosoplastic epithelium by Fluhmann, wherein columnar epithelium is transformed to stratified squamous epithelium. Some of the so-called prosoplastic epithelia may actually represent an essentially normal mode of differentiation restricted to the stratified squamous epithelium in the immediate region of the external os. Because of such juxtaposition, it is attractive to consider that basal or parabasal cells of squamous epithelium grow under a more loosely attached columnar epithelium of the endocervix. In their new environs, these squamous cells enlarge slightly, replicate, and eventually displace overlying columnar epithelium, which degenerates and sluffs off (Fig. 8-11).

CYTOLOGY.—Cells scraped from the squamocolumnar junction may contain varying proportions of squamous, columnar, or reserve cells.

Fig. 8-12.—In the right upper portion of the photomicrograph, there are columnar epithelial cells. To the left, there are numerous reserve cells. The prominent nucleoli reflect a capacity for replication. These cells are morphologically similar to parabasal cells.

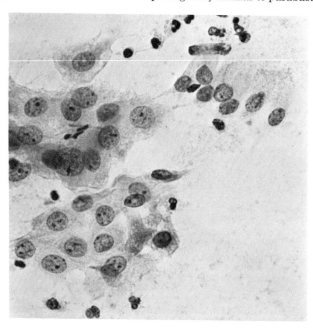

The former two cell types have been described previously. Reserve cells are so commonly seen in cervicovaginal smears that they do not necessarily indicate a pathologic process. They may occur either singly or in small, multicelled clusters. They are relatively small and isodiametric and are similar in size to parabasal cells. The often indistinct cytoplasmic membrane envelops a colorless or very pale blue-green cytoplasm. At times, small, variously sized intracytoplasmic vacuoles may be seen. The almost centrally placed nucleus occupies at least one third of total cell area. It is composed of fine chromatin strands and appears distinctly vesicular; a centrally placed nucleolus is usually present. There may be intercellular bridges. The morphology of these cells is variable, depending on the stage they are in as they transform into mature squamous epithelium (Fig. 8-12).

STROMA—HISTOLOGY[2]

The cervical stroma is composed basically of fibrous connective tissue. As indicated previously, the stroma may contain some smooth muscle fibers, blood vessels, nerves, etc. Stromal elements are only rarely identified in cytologic material.

EMBRYONIC DERIVATIVES—HISTOLOGY

Deep in the lateral wall of the cervix, small tubules lined by low columnar, mucus-positive epithelium with pale cytoplasm and round or oval nuclei may be found.[17] They are remnants of the mesonephric (Wolffian) system and can be observed in up to 40% of histologic sections of the cervix.[16] Such remnants are not seen in cytologic material although they may rarely undergo malignant transformation to clear-cell adenocarcinoma and then exfoliate cells.

REFERENCES

1. Bradburn, G. B., and Webb, C. F.: Cyclic variations in the endocervix, Am. J. Obst. & Gynec. 62:997, 1951.
2. Danforth, D. N.: The fibrous nature of the human cervix, and its relation to the isthmic segment in gravid & non-gravid uteri, Am. J. Obst. & Gynec. 53:541, 1947.
3. Dierks, K.: Der normale mensuelle Ayklus der Menschlichen vaginalschleimhaut, Arch. Gynäk. 130:46, 1927.
4. Fluhmann, C. F.: The squamocolumnar transitional zone of the cervix uteri, Obst. & Gynec. 14:133, 1959.
5. Fluhmann, C. F.: *The Cervix Uteri and Its Diseases* (Philadelphia: W. B. Saunders Company, 1961).
6. Foraker, A. G.: An analysis of nuclear size and nuclear: cytoplasmic ratio in the histological diagnosis of intraepithelial carcinoma of the cervix uteri, Cancer 5:884, 1954.
7. Frost, J. K.: Gynecologic and Obstetric Cytopathology, in Novak: *Gynecologic and Obstetric Pathology* (6th ed.; Philadelphia and London: W. B. Saunders Company, 1967).
8. Graham, C. G.: Uterine cervical epithelium of fetal and immature human females in relation to estrogenic stimulation, Am. J. Obst. & Gynec. 97:1033, 1967.

9. Kaufmann, C., and Ober, K. G.: The Morphological Changes of The Cervix Uteri With Age, and Their Significance in the Early Diagnosis of Carcinoma, in Wolstenholme, G. E. W., and O'Conner, M. (eds.): *Cancer of the Cervix, Diagnosis of Early Forms,* Ciba Foundation Study Group 3 (Boston: Little, Brown & Company, 1959), p. 61.

10. Krantz, K. E., and Phillips, W. P.: Anatomy of the human uterine cervix, gross and microscopic, Ann. New York Acad. Sc., 92:551, 1962.

11. Kury, G., Rev-Kury, L. H., and Friedell, G. H.: Metabolism of human cervical tissues, Am. J. Obst. & Gynec. 98:767, 1967.

12. Laguens, R. P., *et al.*: Fine structure of human endocervical epithelium, Am. J. Obst. & Gynec. 97:1033, 1967.

13. Papanicolaou, G. N.: *Atlas of Exfoliative Cytology* (Cambridge, Mass.: Harvard University Press, 1954).

14. Papanicolaou, G. N., Traut, H. G., and Marchetti, A. A.: *The Epithelial of Woman's Reproductive Organs. A Correlative Study of Cyclic Changes.* (New York: The Commonwealth Fund, 1948).

15. Reagan, J. W., and Ng, A. B. P.: *The Cells of Uterine Adenocarcinoma* (Baltimore: Williams & Wilkins Company, 1965).

16. Sneeden, V. D.: Mesonephric lesions of the cervix. A practical means of demonstration and a suggestion of incidence, Cancer 11:334, 1958.

17. Tiehem, G.: Histogenesis and classification of mesonephric tumors of the female and male genital system and relationship to benign so-called adenomatoid tumors (mesotheliomas). A comparative histological study, Acta path. et microbiol. scandinav. 34:431, 1954.

18. Wied, G. L. (committee chairman): Report by the committee on cytological terminology, in proceedings of the First Internation Congress of Exfoliative Cytology, (Philadelphia and Montreal: J. B. Lippincott Company, 1961), p. 297.

19. Wied, G. L., and Manglano, J. I. A.: Comparative study of the Papanicolaou technique and the acridine-orange fluorescence method, Acta cytol. 6:554, 1962.

20. Opinion poll on cytologic definition, Acta cytol. 2:25, 1958.

CHAPTER 9

Squamous Dysplasia

THE TERM DYSPLASIA is used to describe a broad spectrum of lesions and is defined only with great difficulty. Compounding the difficulty of definition is a plethora of synonyms. They include such terms as dyskeratosis,[17] atypical hyperplasia,[17] atypia, benign atypia, simple atypical epithelium, irregular and increasingly atypical epithelium, squamous metaplasia with atypicality, anaplasia, precancerous metaplasia, dissociated intraepithelial anaplasia, basal cell hyperplasia or hyperactivity, dyskaryosis, leukohyperkeratosis and leukoparakeratosis.[11] The cytohistologic changes of dysplasia sometimes reflect the influence of known exogenous factors, whereas in others the agent is unknown. Accordingly, they are classifiable as primary or secondary dysplasia (Table 9-1).

Both experimental and clinical examples of "exogenous dysplasia" have been described. Patten and associates[8] were able to induce such a change in 22% of young adult, female mice following weekly intravaginal introduction of *Trichomonas vaginalis*. The reaction disappeared following removal of the organism. However, the causative role of *Trichomonas vaginalis* in dysplasia in the human has not been elucidated. Such an association is doubtful,[1, 6] and a cause-and-effect relationship is difficult to prove because of antigenic strain differences among trichomonads. It is commonly accepted that *Trichomonas vaginalis* may cause such cellular alterations as perinuclear halos, cytoplasmic eosinophilia, slight nuclear and cellular enlargement, binucleation and nuclear pyknosis of squamous cells, but abnormalities cytologically representative of dysplasia have not been observed in humans (Fig. 9-1). Administration of alkylating agents, such as busulfan (Myleran), has been associated with cytologic changes simulating dysplasia[5, 18] (see Fig. 20-12, *A* and *B*). Apparently such alterations are not reversible following cessation of therapy.[5] Other circumstances, such as silver nitrate cauterization,[2] podophyllin administration[4] or intravaginal painting with methylcholanthrene in mice,[21] may induce lesions indistinquishable cytologically and/or histologically from dysplasia. Cellular changes induced by podophyllin commence approximately 24 hours after local

73

TABLE 9-1.—Dysplasia Classification

Primary	Secondary
In nongravid women	Trichomonas
In gravid women	Alkylating agents
Following radiation Rx	Silver nitrate cautery
	Podophyllin
	Methylcholanthrene
	IUD
	Squamous papillomas
	Repair processes

application.[15] The alterations are reversible; in animals they have been noted to disappear within 5 days after discontinuance of the drug.[16] The relationship of intrauterine devices (IUD) to the incidence and progression of dysplasia has been variously reported; obviously, evaluation of the significance of IUD's is difficult (Fig. 9-2). For example, most women wearing such devices will be multiparous, thereby representing a population with a relatively high incidence of dysplasia. A study of women with dysplasia using IUD's and a similar control group not using IUD's showed no carcinogenic effect of these devices.[14] Similarly, the rate of progression of dysplasia to in situ cancer did not differ in groups of patients with and without IUD's.[14] The IUD may, however, induce markedly hyperplastic squamous or glandular changes that are reversible following removal of the device. Squamous papillomas (condylomata acuminata) of the female genital tract, possibly of viral etiology, are usually associated with a cytologic picture mimicking dysplasia (Fig. 9-3). Similarly, individual cells from repair processes, or decidual cells,

Fig. 9-1.—Trichomonas change. Cells present in the trichomonas change are generally eosinophilic, occur singly, **A** or in groups, **B**. They may exhibit nuclear enlargement with hyperchromasia and are generally isodiametric. The most characteristic diagnostic features, however, are "perinuclear halos" (*arrows*, **A**), cytoplasmic eosinophilia, and nuclear pyknosis. In addition to the presence of the protozoan parasite *Trichomonas vaginalis*, inflammatory cells in the form of polymorphonuclear leukocytes are invariably present, except for selected cases. It is necessary to be conversant with the trichomonas change so that an incorrect diagnosis of dysplasia is not rendered.

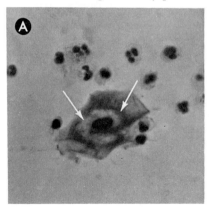
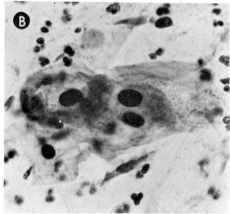

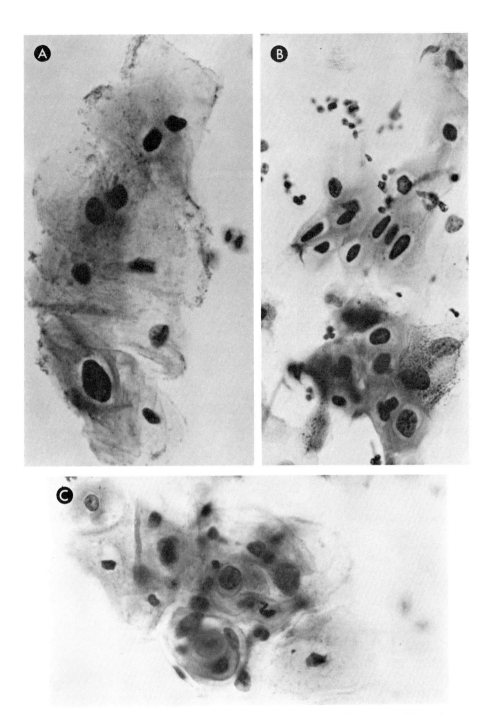

Fig. 9-2.—Cells from a cervical smear of a woman who had a loop inserted into the uterine cavity. Following removal of the loop the cellular changes regressed markedly. **A** and **B**, while showing certain similarities to cells of dysplasia, these cells probably represent a cervical erosion secondary to the string attached to the loop. For example, they have an eosinophilic cytoplasm, are often irregular and, as seen in **C**, are arranged in benign pearl formations. When mild atypia, as shown here, is associated with a potential causative factor such as a loop or trichomonads, we often suggest removal or treatment of that factor followed by a repeat smear. This enables us to weed out non-neoplastic conditions simulating dysplasia.

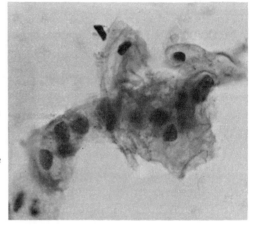

Fig. 9-3. – Cells from a patient with a condylomata acuminata (squamous papilloma) of the cervix. Many characteristics of dysplastic cells are evident, so that differentiation of these two conditions is often impossible by purely cytologic means.

may simulate dysplastic cells (Fig. 9-4; also see Figs. 20-10, *A* and *B*). The general cytologic pattern in cases suggestive of dysplasia must be evaluated with great care and correlated with the pertinent history. In addition, we often recommend repeat smears in such instances immediately following elimination of a known inciting agent, or after treatment of "cervicitis." In most cases of dysplasia, however, inciting factors are unknown.

The lesion called dysplasia commences as a more profoundly disturbing epithelial alteration than any seen in ordinary repair processes. The alteration comprises a broad spectrum, stopping just short of carcinoma in situ. Specific criteria for the diagnosis in situ cancer are difficult to establish; thus, the more malignant end of the spectrum is also somewhat blurred. Accordingly, both the cytologic and the histologic

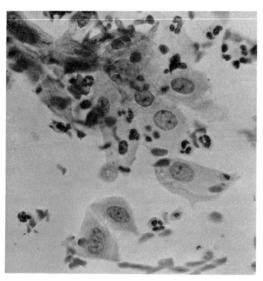

Fig. 9-4. – Cells representing a repair process. The enlarged nuclei are not hyperchromatic and contain nucleoli, both features uncommon in dysplastic cells. See Figure 20-10.

diagnoses of dysplasia are often beset with insurmountable difficulties. When the cytologic findings suggesting dysplasia are minimal, conservative interpretation is indicated. Repetition of the smear rather than immediate biopsy is advocated. On the other hand, when the cytologic findings approach the features of in situ cancer, biopsy is indicated as the more definitive approach. Even should an initial punch biopsy "confirm" the presence of dysplasia, it should not be assumed that the maximum alteration has been demonstrated. For example, Varga[17] showed that, of 78 patients in whom the initial cervical punch biopsy revealed dysplasia, subsequent study established the diagnosis of carcinoma in situ in 39 and invasive cancer in 11. Dysplasia may be seen in both gravid and nongravid women, or following radiotherapy for cervical squamous cancer (see Chap. 19). It is advisable to segregate those groups from others, since the lesion may manifest a different biologic potential in such instances. The variable incidences of various types of dysplasia are discussed in applicable sections.

Dysplasia Not Associated With Pregnancy or Postirradiation

The biologic behavior of dysplasia, unassociated with pregnancy, is currently disputed by investigators representing two different schools of thought. The first is that dysplasia demonstrates variable and unpredictable behavior; the lesion may regress, remain stable or progress to in situ cancer. Others propose that the true dysplastic reaction, whether in the presence or absence of pregnancy, is not reversible, but may remain stable or, less frequently, progress to some form of cancer.[12] It is self-evident that the alleged disappearance of dysplasia inherent in the first hypothesis may result from the curative effects of diagnostic biopsy; in the course of such biopsy, the entire dysplastic lesion might be removed. In view of the difficulty of evaluating the validity of either theory, the final answer to the dilemma must await the wisdom of time.

Usually, there are fewer altered cells in smears from patients with dysplasia than in those from patients with carcinoma in situ,[7, 10] although variation exists in given instances. This feature of dysplasia probably reflects the increased cohesiveness of the cells forming the dysplastic lesion, as well as the smaller size of the dysplastic lesion on the exposed portion of the cervix when compared to those of in situ cancer.[13] However, dysplastic cells in smear preparations almost always appear singly or in small groupings with visible cell borders. The shape of the cells is usually polyhedral, although some may be oval, round or ellipsoidal (Figs. 9-5 and 9-6). Irregular cell types and syncytial groupings, common in smears from invasive cancers, are only rarely encountered. The cells of dysplasia are slightly smaller in average size than normal intermediate cells, which rarely contain vacuoles; tinctorial

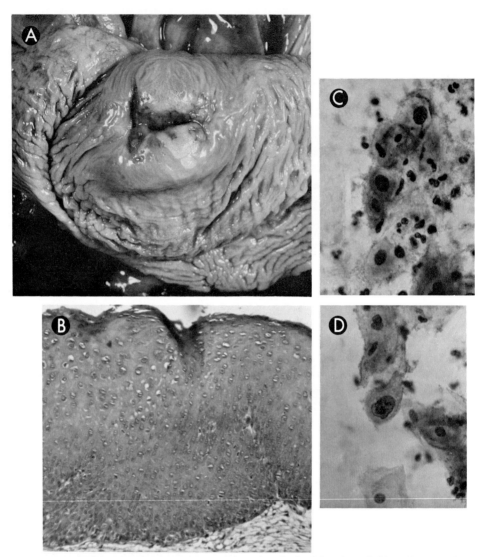

Fig. 9-5. — Mild dysplasia in a 14-year-old female who had her first child at the age of 13 and died at 16 from sniffing glue. **A,** gross appearance of the cervix at autopsy. Note the whitish area which corresponds to the findings depicted in the tissue photomicrograph (**B**). **B,** tissue photomicrograph. A thin layer of anucleated squamous cells overlie, representing associated leukoplakia. This lesion may be considered leukokeratosis by some. **C** and **D,** characteristic isolated cells which are generally isodiametric, and have slightly enlarged nuclei with hyperchromasia.

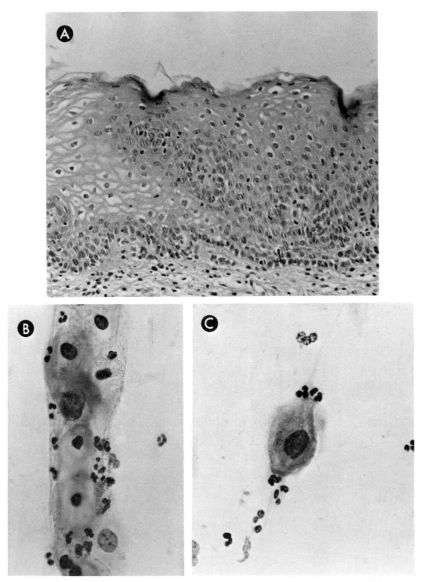

Fig. 9-6. – Proven mild dysplasia. **A**, tissue photomicrograph of the cervical biopsy. Note the normal squamous epithelium to the left with the abrupt transition to mildly dysplastic epithelium on the right. The junction between normal and atypical epithelium is called *the line of Schiller*. **B** and **C**, cells from the patient. Abnormal cells were few in number and showed the usual findings of dysplasia.

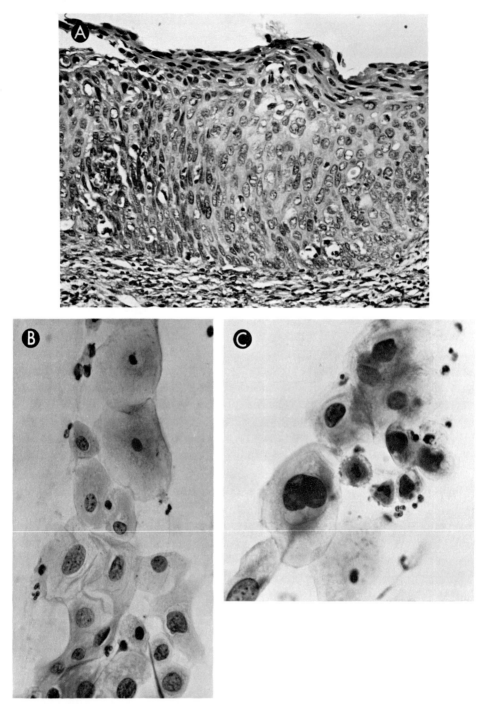

Fig. 9-7.—Classic marked dysplasia. **A,** tissue photomicrograph of the cervical biopsy. As the cells reach the luminal border they tend to become parallel to the plane of endocervical canal. **B** and **C,** cells. Note the variation from fairly large dysplastic cells to a few that are smaller and more closely resemble isodiametric parabasal cells of in situ cancer. When the latter cell type is present in fairly large numbers, the presence of in situ cancer is likely.

qualities of dysplastic cells, like intermediate cells seen during pregnancy, are generally cyanophilic and, less commonly, eosinophilic. The usually encountered oval or round nuclei may at times be multiple or irregular in shape (Fig. 9-7). The nuclei are significantly larger than those of cells of in situ cancer, but nevertheless occupy a proportionately smaller area of the cell (15% vs. 32%). Nuclei reveal a variable chromatin pattern, usually hyperchromatic, uniform and finely granular, or, less commonly, opaque with coarse, chromatin strands, due to irregular deposition of chromatinic material. Nucleoli are so rarely encountered that, should they be present in an appreciable number of cells, a diagnosis of dysplasia is highly unlikely.

Dysplasia Associated With Pregnancy

Not only is dysplasia more common during pregnancy but it is more frequent with increasing parity.[11] Dysplasia in pregnancy occurs most often in the age range at which pregnancy attains its maximal frequency—the middle and late third decade. We observed an age range of 13 to 42 years and our patients had an average of 4.3 pregnancies (range 1–13), with a mean age of 17 years at the time of their first pregnancy. One-third had nonspecific symptoms, such as bleeding or mucoid discharge. It is not always possible to determine whether or not a dysplastic lesion antedates or originates during pregnancy (Figs. 9-8 and 9-9). However, when diagnosed during pregnancy, the lesion often persists after delivery, although it may disappear during pregnancy or in the early postpartum period. At times, progression to in situ cancer may occur (Fig. 9-10). Of 28 women with dysplasia in pregnancy, Reagan and associates observed that in 14 the lesion persisted after delivery; in 9 of them, it remained present for varying periods of time. Those with persistent disease generally had a higher initial dysplastic cell count than those without persistent disease. This suggests that smaller lesions may be "cured" by the trauma of delivery.[3, 20] Cervical lacerations, bruising or erosions occur more frequently in primiparas (97%), although they are no stranger to multiparas (58%). By 6 weeks post partum, most traumatic lesions will have healed.[20] It is possible that there may be abnormal healing of those postpartum changes. In transformation or mosaic zones,[12, 13] abnormal cells may often be seen, perhaps initiating a new or perpetuating a prior disease process.[19]

The cytomorphology of dysplastic cells in pregnancy does not ordinarily differ significantly from those seen in the nongravid state. Several features of dysplastic cells, while more commonly seen in the pregnant patient,[11] are of questionable diagnostic value in any individual instance. Such changes include a smaller cell size earlier in pregnancy, with increase as pregnancy advances. The cytoplasm is generally more

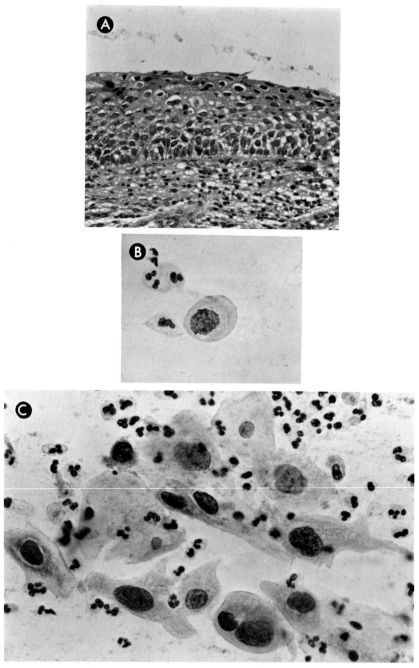

Fig. 9-8.—Moderate dysplasia during pregnancy. **A,** tissue photomicrograph of the biopsy. This lesion did not regress following delivery and carcinoma in situ eventually occurred. **B** and **C,** typical cyanophilic, moderately dysplastic cells observed. The cells are generally isodiametric and contain modestly enlarged, hyperchromatic nuclei. Binucleation can be observed.

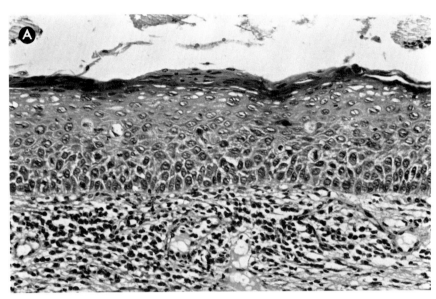

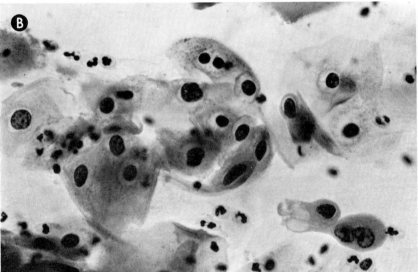

Fig. 9-9. — Further study of the patient whose cells and biopsy are shown in Figure 9-8. It was discovered that moderate dysplasia antedated her pregnancy. Comparison of the biopsy tissue photomicrograph, **A**, and the cells, **B**, with Figure 9-8 shows similar findings before and during pregnancy, although the dysplastic cells seen in **B** were slightly enlarged during pregnancy. Pregnancy probably has little effect on an existing dysplastic process and many dysplasias initially diagnosed during pregnancy are, in reality, carryovers from a condition present before pregnancy.

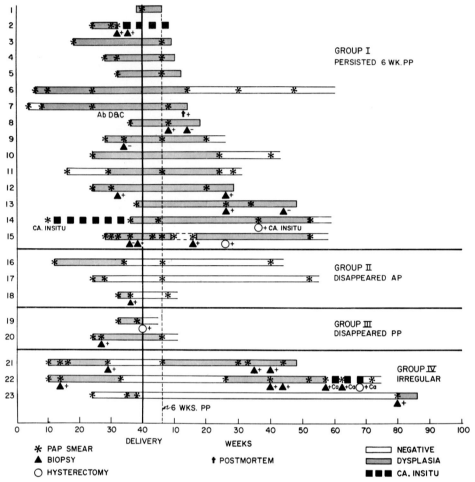

Fig. 9-10. — Fate of dysplasia diagnosed during pregnancy.

vacuolated during pregnancy; nuclear mass is larger in early than in late pregnancy.[9, 10, 11] Among the dysplastic cell population of pregnancy, presence of multiple nuclei has been reported in 5.2%, whereas, in those not pregnant,[9] only 3% of dysplastic cells are multinucleated.[9]

REFERENCES

1. Hulka, B. S., and Hulka, J. F.: Dyskaryosis in cervical cytology and its relationship to trichomoniasis therapy, Am. J. Obst. & Gynec. 98:180, 1967.
2. Hulka, J. F., and Ison, A.: Silver nitrate and cervical cytology, Am. J. Obst. & Gynec. 90:1361, 1964.
3. Johnson, L. D., Sheps, M. C., and Easterday, C. L.: The cervix in pregnancy and the postpartum period I. The correlation of certain clinical factors with the clinical appearance of the cervix, Obst. & Gynec. 14:452, 1959.
4. Kaminetzky, H. A., and Sberlow, M.: Podophyllin and the mouse cervix: assessment of carcinogenic potential, Am. J. Obst. & Gynec. 93:486, 1965.
5. Koss, L. G., Melamed, M. R., and Mayer, K.: The effect of busulfan on human epithelia, Am. J. Clin. Path. 44:385, 1965.

6. Koss, L. G., and Wolinska, W. H.: Trichomonas vaginalis cervicitis and its relationship to cervical cancer. A histocytological study, Cancer 12:1171, 1959.

7. Okagaki, T., *et al.*: Diagnosis of anaplasia and carcinoma in situ by differential cell counts, Acta cytol. 6:343, 1962.

8. Patten, S. F., Jr., Hughes, C. P., and Reagan, J. W.: An experimental study of the relationship between *Trichomonas vaginalis* and dysplasia in the uterine cervix, Acta cytol. 7:187, 1963.

9. Reagan, J. W., Seidemann, I. L., and Patten, S. F., Jr.: Developmental stages of in situ carcinoma in uterine cervix: an analytical study of the cells, Acta cytol. 6:538, 1962.

10. Reagan, J. W., Seidemann, I. L., and Saracusa, Y.: The cellular morphology of carcinoma in situ and dysplasia or atypical hyperplasia of the uterine cervix, Cancer 6:224, 1953.

11. Reagan, J. W., *et al.*: Dysplasia in the uterine cervix during pregnancy: an analytical study of the cells, Acta cytol. 5:17, 1961.

12. Richart, R. M.: Cervical neoplasia in pregnancy. A series of pregnant and postpartum patients followed without biopsy or therapy, Am. J. Obst. & Gynec. 87:474, 1963.

13. Richart, R. M.: Colpomicroscopic studies of the distribution of dysplasia and carcinoma in situ on the exposed portion of the human uterine cervix, Cancer 18:950, 1965.

14. Richart, R. M., and Barron, B. A.: The intrauterine device and cervical neoplasia. A prospective study of patients with cervical dysplasia, J.A.M.A. 199:817, 1967.

15. Saphir, O., Leventhal, M. L., and Kline, T. S.: Podophyllin-induced dysplasia of the cervix uteri: its histologic resemblance to carcinoma in situ, Am. J. Clin. Path. 32:446, 1959.

16. Standish, S. M., and Schafer, W. G.: Effects of podophyllin on epithelial tissues, Arch. Path. 72:48, 1961.

17. Varga, A.: The relationship of cervical dysplasia to in situ and invasive carcinoma of the cervix, Am. J. Obst. & Gynec. 95:759, 1966.

18. Ward, H. N., Konikov, M., and Reinhard, E. H.: Cytologic dysplasia occurring after busulfan (Myleran) therapy, Ann. Int. Med. 63:654, 1965.

19. Wilbanks, G. D., and Richart, R. M.: Postpartum cervix and its relation to cervical neoplasia, Cancer 19:273, 1966.

20. Wilbanks, G. D., and Richart, R. M.: The puerperal cervix, injuries and healing, Am. J. Obst. & Gynec. 97:1105, 1967.

21. Yang, Y. H., and Campbell, J. S.: Evolution of dysplasia of the uterine cervix and vagina induced by low doses of carcinogen in mice, Obst. & Gynec. 26:91, 1965.

CHAPTER 10

The Cytopathology of Squamous Carcinoma In Situ of the Cervix Uteri

The Concept

CELLULAR "SPREADS"

MODERN CYTODIAGNOSIS no longer depends primarily on the study of exfoliated material. Instead, its basis is the study of cells scraped directly or aspirated from areas near to those suspected of harboring a neoplasm. The specimen applied to a slide is in essence a tissue spread or "microbiopsy." If the technique has been adequate, the "spread" should be a good representation of surface cells from the area of collection. By studying the various cellular patterns present, it is possible to determine whether or not malignancy is present. Commonly, it is possible to translate that information to indicate accurately a specific diagnosis conforming to tissue findings. The study of spontaneously exfoliated cells is ordinarily inferior to the just-mentioned collection method. Because spontaneous desquamation usually occurs from many areas, a dilution factor accompanies which may compromise the malignant cell population. In contrast, innumerable malignant cells are commonly encountered when there has been a direct scrape.

CELL NUMBERS AND THE CANCER TREND

As suggested in the preceding section, accuracy in the cytologic prediction of carcinoma in situ of the cervix is roughly proportional to the number of malignant cells encountered. Proper collection techniques in that disease can be expected to yield many malignant cells. For example, Reagan and Hamonic demonstrated that patients with in situ cancer can be expected to have 500 or more malignant cells in over 75% of cases by the cellular spread method.[18] Obviously, if a lesion is located on the portio, a cervical scrape will produce more malignant cells, while canal neoplasms are more susceptible to diagnosis by endocervical aspiration. In that regard, it is important to remember that older patients often have in situ cancer located high in the endocervical canal, further emphasizing the necessity of the endocervical aspiration. If only a few malignant cells are discovered after careful screening, we feel that it is advisable to obtain immediate fractionated specimens, i.e., vaginal pool, cervical scrape and endocervical aspiration, marked accordingly. By such means, a more precise cytologic evaluation is possible, often with an indication of the most probable location of the suspected lesion.

Under ordinary conditions, smears from a patient with in situ cancer of the cervix contain a spectrum of cells ranging from those that are benign to those of undoubted malignant nature. The cell distribution exhibits a certain predictability. For example, slightly over 50% of them will be normal, about 15% dysplastic, and about 35% malignant, conforming primarily to the type seen in carcinoma in situ. In contrast, dysplasia has a population almost exclusively of normal and dysplastic cells, in varying proportions. Smears from invasive cancer have fewer normal and dysplastic but more malignant elements than in situ cancer; the malignant cells conform less to those seen in carcinoma in situ and more so to undifferentiated cancer cells.

Individual Cell Specificity

The morphologic appearance of a single cell can rarely be depended upon to indicate accurately its biologic potentiality. Thus it is inadvisable to attempt a definitive diagnosis in such a circumstance. For example, cell elements that are fiber-like, mitotic, in pearls, with naked nuclei, syncytial, clustered, hyperchromatic, degenerated or irregular can be observed in both benign and malignant disease or, at times, in disease-free patients. Even biologic activity, determined by thymidine turnover, is not a decisive differentiating feature as normal basal cells, those partaking in repair and malignant neoplastic ones may have remarkably similar activity. Chromosome analysis may be useful to detect abnormalities (aneuploidy, polyploidy or, at times, euploidy) among groups or clones of malignant cells. Unfortunately, at times only a very small percentage of cells of in situ cancer may show aneuploidy and, in the last analysis, chromosome study is of no practical diagnostic value in that disease.[24, 28]

Characteristics of Cells Seen in Carcinoma in Situ

Despite obvious morphologic overlap between certain cells that are benign and those of in situ cancer, certain general characteristics (cell arrangement, size and configuration) are common among the latter.

General Cellular Characteristics

CELL ARRANGEMENT. — The cells of in situ cancer usually have decreased adhesiveness between mutual members. Consequently, if cytologic smears are studied from a vaginal pool specimen, the malignant cells usually occur singly. However, study of cells from a surface that has been scraped will often result in a significant number of cells that appear in clusters, i.e., cells are directly apposed to one another with cell membranes being recognizable.[22, 30] This has been likened to a "microbiopsy" (Fig. 10-1).[22]

Reagan and Hamonic[18] noted in carcinoma in situ that 72.08% of cells were isolated whereas 27.92% were in groups. Wied *et al.*[30] reported similar findings. Our observations indicate that cell clustering may be even more commonly seen and prevails to a greater extent in material collected from women under 50 years of age. In many of the aforementioned cell groupings, it is difficult to define cell borders precisely, but the fairly even disposition of nuclei is suggestive that they are not truly syncytial. This contrasts with commonly observed syncytial cells in smears from invasive cancer.[21, 30] Some believe that most cell groups in carcinoma in situ are actually syncytial.[22]

Fig. 10-1. — Smear containing a large group of malignant cells scraped from the cervix of a patient with carcinoma in situ (CIS). Such large clusters may be likened to a "microbiopsy."

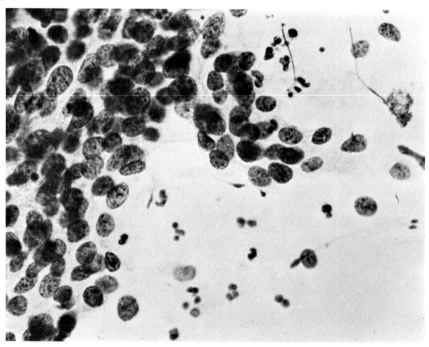

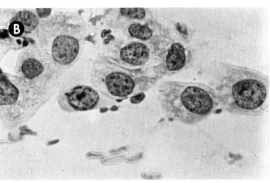

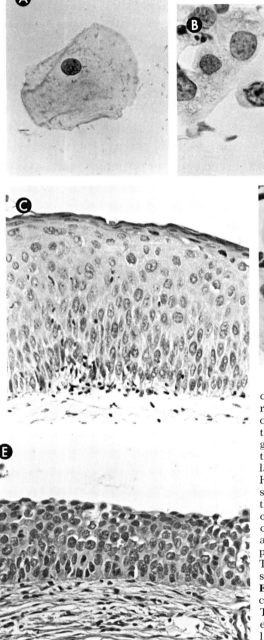

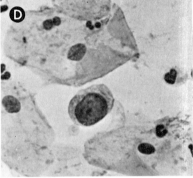

Fig. 10-2. – Cells in dysplasia and carcinoma in situ (CIS). **A**, representative normal intermediate cell. Note that it is larger than those of dysplasia (**B**) or CIS (**D**). **B**, groups of dysplastic cells. Note that the cell and nuclear areas are larger than the cells of CIS (**D**). However, dysplastic cells show smaller nuclear/cytoplasmic ratios than CIS cells. **C**, photomicrograph of the tissue counterpart of the classic dysplastic cells seen in **B**. H. and E. ×64. **D**, a malignant parabasal cell characteristic of CIS. Total cell and nuclear area is smaller than in dysplastic cells (**B**). **E**, photomicrograph of the tissue counterpart of the cells seen in **D**. The malignant parabasal cells extend through the entire epithelial layer. H. and E. ×64.

CELL SIZE.—In general, the cells of in situ cancer are distinctly smaller than normal superficial or intermediate epithelial elements.[22] The neoplastic cells correspond closely in size to those that are basal (germinative), parabasal or reserve. However, some malignant cells of in situ cancer are similar in size to normal intermediate cells, in which instances they are predominantly non-isodiametric, i.e., large-cell keratinizing and undifferentiated cells. For the most part, the size of cells of in situ cancer is a reflection of the size of the parent cell, which they mimic in their relatively well-differentiated state. The cells in dysplasia and invasive cancer are generally larger and smaller, respectively, than those of in situ malignancy (Fig. 10-2).[22]

CELL CONFIGURATION.—The cells of in situ cancer are characteristically isodiametric as polyhedral, oval or round forms.[18, 30] Such cellular elements predominate in women less than 50 years of age. However, those over 50 commonly have forms that are irregular, characteristically with keratinizing cytoplasm. At times, in situ cancer may have fiber cells. They probably originate from the surface, a result of pressure effects from underlying cells on one side and the endocervical canal on the other. Tadpole shapes are so uncommon in smears from in situ cancer that their presence is highly suspicious of the existence of an invasive malignancy. In general, irregular cell forms are much commoner in invasive cancer.

CYTOPLASMIC CHARACTERISTICS

CYTOPLASMIC COLOR.—Most malignant cells from the female genital tract have a cytoplasm that stains either light blue-green or is colorless. Keratinizing cancer cells which may be seen in either carcinoma in situ or invasive cancer are an important exception. The keratinizing cancer cell type represents less than 10% of the cell population of in situ cancer in younger patients (less than 50) but may account for almost one half of the cells from the same lesion in older women.

CYTOPLASMIC INCLUSIONS.—Cytoplasmic vacuoles are rarely a conspicuous feature of the cells of in situ cancer, although in that disease vacuoles are more commonly encountered than in the invasive counterpart. Some degree of localized or diffuse cytoplasmic vacuolization has been noted in about 10% of cells in carcinoma in situ.[18] It is possible that such cells originated from reserve (or prosoplastic) cells, which are commonly finely vacuolated. At times, polymorphonuclear leukocytes may be intracytoplasmic in carcinoma in situ. However, they are more commonly seen in invasive squamous and adenocarcinoma. The presence of such inflammatory cells is most likely a reaction to early cell death.

CELL MEMBRANE.—A well-defined cell membrane is unusual but it is more prominent with less anaplasia.

NUCLEAR CHARACTERISTICS

CHROMATIN PATTERN OF THE NUCLEUS. — Nuclear chromatin patterns in cancer in situ are variable and may be finely granular (Fig. 10-3, *A*), coarsely granular or almost opaque (Fig. 10-3, *B* and *C*).[19] Cells from in situ cancer usually have nuclei that are coarsely granular (Fig. 10-4). However, nuclear chromatinic material does not necessarily increase in amount relative to the severity of the lesion, i.e., when comparing dysplasia, in situ cancer and invasive squamous cell carcinoma. Lindner[12]

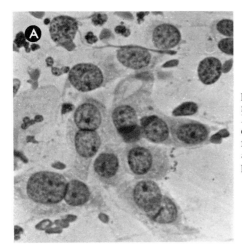

Fig. 10-3. — Nuclear chromatic patterns in patients with CIS. **A**, finely granular pattern in cells from a smear. In some cells there are chromocenters, or nucleoli. **B** and **C**, cells in a smear from two patients which demonstrate an almost opaque nuclear chromatin pattern.

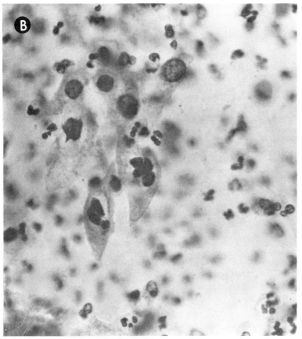

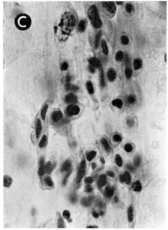

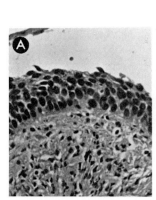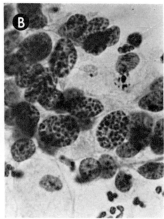

Fig. 10-4. – Nuclei in cells of patients with CIS. **A**, histologic section showing coarsely granular nuclei. **B**, cells in a smear from the same patient as **A**. They contain nuclei with the coarsely granular chromatin pattern that is the commonest pattern in cells of in situ cancer.

has suggested that nuclear staining characteristics of carcinoma in situ are due to changes associated with beginning death of these cells. The recent cell death leads to further increase in nuclear size with chromatin clumping. The various nuclear chromatin patterns in carcinoma in situ are detailed under the heading, "Specific Cell Types Seen in Carcinoma In Situ" on pages 94 to 102.

NUCLEAR CONFIGURATION. – Nuclear configuration in carcinoma in situ is usually regular, the constituent cells having round-to-oval nuclei. Certain cells seen in cancer in situ may have irregular nuclear configurations, i.e., keratinizing and undifferentiated cancer cells. Nuclei of the small cell variety of in situ cancer are rounded, but careful inspection almost always demonstrates areas of irregularity. Elongate nuclei are characteristic in fiber cells, not uncommonly observed in cancer in situ. However, elongate or irregular nuclear forms are found in greater numbers in invasive malignancy.[22]

NUCLEAR SIZE. – Absolute nuclear areas of normal squamous cells are significantly smaller than those of dysplasia, in situ cancer, and invasive cancer. In general, mean nuclear areas progressively decrease in size from dysplasia to in situ cancer and, lastly, to invasive malignancy. It is worthwhile to note that some non-neoplastic conditions have cells with markedly enlarged nuclei. They include those associated with healing, following radiation therapy, in megaloblastic anemias and reacting to various inflammatory stimuli such as chronic cervicitis. Nuclear areas alone are relatively unimportant compared to the significance of the relationship of nuclear area to over-all cell size.

NUCLEAR/CYTOPLASMIC RATIO. – A fairly dependable feature of the

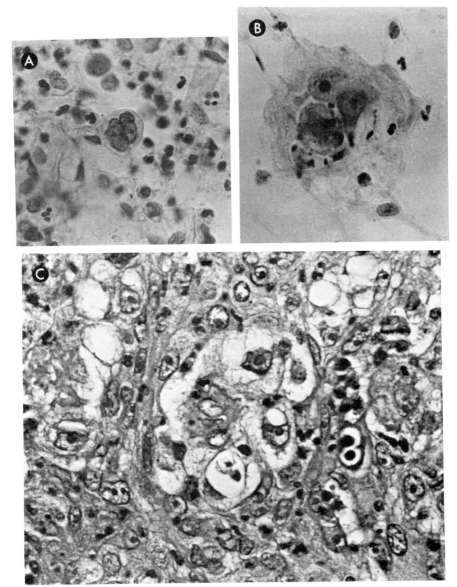

Fig. 10-5. – Multinucleation. **A**, a binucleated cell in a smear from a patient with CIS. Multinucleation is frequently encountered in smears from patients with dysplasia or invasive cancer. **B**, a syncytial, multinucleated cell in a smear from a patient with invasive cancer of the cervix. Nucleoli are apparent in some cells. Both multinucleation and the presence of nucleoli are encountered more commonly in cells representative of invasive cancer. **C**, a histologic section of the cervix of the patient in **B**, which contains invasive large, nonkeratinizing squamous cell cancer. H. and E. ×160.

malignant cell is the nuclear/cytoplasmic ratio. It is usually expressed as a fraction representing the relative nuclear area. The cells of squamous in situ cancer have nuclei that occupy almost 14 times more cell area than normal superficial squamous elements.[22, 30] Johnston[8] noted that 70% of cells from invasive squamous cancer and 80% from in situ cancers had cytoplasmic/nuclear ratios less than 3.5. Most normal cells, except those of basal or parabasal origin, had higher ratios. In general, more advanced lesions (i.e., invasive squamous cancer) have slightly greater relative nuclear areas although the absolute nuclear areas decrease.[2, 18, 22] Such comparisons are only valid when made between cells of identical parent origin. For example, the mean nuclear area of a normal cervical columnar cell and a malignant squamous one may be in agreement.[20, 22, 30] However, even certain normal constituents of a given area may demonstrate large nuclear/cytoplasmic ratios, such as cells of parabasal origin in aged patients and following radiotherapy.[8] Basal cells have similar large nuclear/cytoplasmic ratio characteristics but are not ordinarily observed in cytologic material. Such benign cell types are readily differentiated by their benign nuclear structure.

MULTINUCLEATION.—Multinucleation is an inconstant feature in cellular preparations from carcinoma in situ (Fig. 10-5, A). Reagan and Hamonic[18] found 1.4% of cells studied from in situ lesions were multinucleated, containing from two to seven nuclei. Multinucleated cells are somewhat more commonly observed in material from those with dysplasia but are much more frequent from those with invasive squamous cancer (Fig. 10-5, B and C). Multinucleated cells are commonly encountered in cytologic material from people with non-neoplastic conditions. For example, they are often associated with chronic cervicitis, herpes genitalis, radiation or radiomimetic drug therapy, pregnancy (syncytiotrophoblast) and, at times, megaloblastic anemias.

NUCLEOLI.—Nucleoli are occasionally seen in cells from in situ cancer (Fig. 10-3, A). Reagan and Hamonic[18] found them in 4.77% of counted cells and in a little over half of their cases. We have noted that when nucleoli are present, associated nuclear chromatinic material is often finely dispersed. Such cells strongly resemble those of adenocarcinoma and are often arranged in sheets. Dysplastic cells rarely have nucleoli, whereas those from invasive squamous cancer are much more commonly nucleolated than cells representative of in situ cancer. Nucleoli are a characteristic feature in cells of benign and malignant glandular origin, decidua, healing ulcers, histiocytes, stromal and reserve cells.

Specific Cell Types Seen in Carcinoma In Situ

The malignant cell population of in situ cancer is variously composed of eight cell types, as follows:

MALIGNANT PARABASAL CELL (third-type cell of Graham[3, 4]).—These

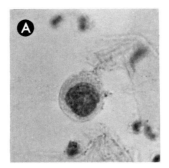

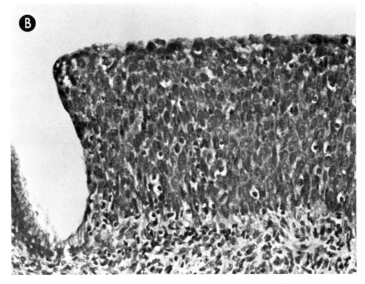

Fig. 10-6. — Malignant parabasal cells. **A,** a rather typical isodiametric malignant parabasal cell in a smear from a patient with CIS. The nuclear chromatin is coarsely clumped.
Cytoplasmic and nuclear configurations are usually round, oval, or ellipsoidal and the
cytoplasm is most commonly cyanophilic. Nuclei seldom occupy less than ½ of the total
cell area. **B,** histologic section evidencing the classic appearance of in situ cancer. The
stroma has not been invaded; there is a definite loss of polarity of cells from the basal layer to the luminal border of the epithelium; and individual cells show malignant characteristics. H. and E. ×64.

cells represent the commonest cell type seen in cancer in situ (Fig. 10-6).
They are generally the size of an inner basal cell and are round or oval.
The nucleus occupies a large area with the distance from the nuclear
border to the cellular border being less than the maximum diameter of
the nucleus. The nuclear chromatin shows variable degrees of clumping
but is rarely either vesicular* or "India ink"† in character. Nucleoli will
occasionally be observed. The cytoplasm is usually basophilic but may
stain variably.[4]

---

*In this context, the term *vesicular* refers to spaces in the nucleus that fail to stain
with hematoxylin.

†"India ink" nuclei stain intensely with hematoxylin and are black, homogeneous and
opaque.

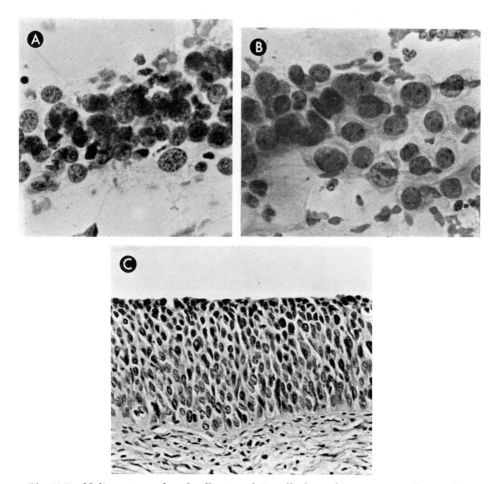

Fig. 10-7.—Malignant parabasal cells. **A** and **B**, cells from this smear are clustered, so-called clustered cancer cells. When cells are removed by forcibly scraping the cervix, parabasal cells are more commonly encountered in groupings. The grouping in **A** is probably syncytial, while the cells in **B** are in apposition one to the other with recognized cell borders. Note the erythrocytes in **A**, a common finding in smears from patients with cancer in situ. **C**, a histologic section corresponding to the cytology depicted in **A** and **B**. The epithelial pattern is in all respects similar to that in Fig. 10-6*B*. H. and E. ×64.

CLUSTERED CANCER CELL.—These cells are quite similar to the description for the malignant parabasal type cell just noted. In fact, they strongly resemble clustered parabasals and are often shaped in non-isodiametric patterns (Fig. 10-7). Such shapes are created by pressure effects of the surrounding cells and may be noted in tissue sections of carcinoma in situ. At times it may be difficult to recognize cell borders between individual cells in a cluster. However, because of fairly even nuclear dispersion, they are possibly not part of a syncytium. Nuclear and cytoplasmic features generally parallel those of third-type cells.[3]

LARGE NONKERATINIZING CELL.—These round or oval cells may be

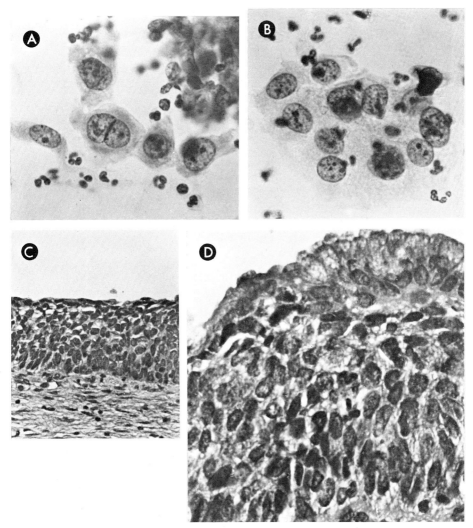

Fig. 10-8.—Nonkeratinizing cancer cells. **A** and **B**, photomicrographs of cells in a smear from a patient with CIS. Nuclei of these usually isodiametric cells often contain nucleoli and have vesicular zones. Cell groupings are encountered so commonly that, when combined with the feature of prominent nucleoli, differentiation from cells of adenocarcinoma is difficult. **C** and **D**, histologic sections of the carcinoma in situ of the cervix of the patient whose cells are depicted in **A** and **B**. The over-all pattern is similar to that depicted in Figures 10-2*E*, 10-4*B*, 10-6*B* and 10-7*C*. This lesion, however, is more often encountered beneath overlying endocervical columnar epithelium. H. and E. **C** × 64, **D** × 160.

larger or smaller than the parabasal-type cell. They may also display modest irregularity. The mean nuclear area is greater than that of parabasal-type cells and the nucleus generally has irregularly granular, stippled chromatin pattern with frequent vesicular areas. Nucleoli are often conspicuous, not unlike the pattern seen in cells of adenocarcinoma (Fig. 10-8). To further accentuate their resemblance to cells of glandu-

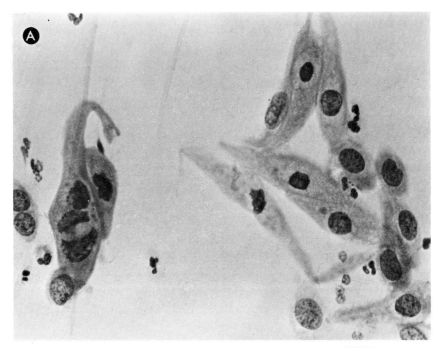

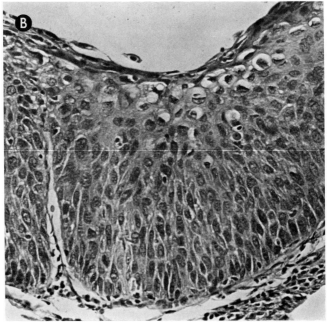

Fig. 10-9. – Keratinizing cancer cells. **A,** cells in a smear from a patient with CIS. Such cells are characteristically irregular and have eosinophilic cytoplasm. Irregular nuclei have a coarsely clumped to opaque chromatin pattern. Malignant fiber cells or anucleate squames (due to commonly associated leukoplakia) are often seen. **B,** histologic section of the keratinizing variety of in situ cancer. This photomicrograph corresponds to the cytology shown in **A.** The irregularity of constituent cells forming the lesion is readily observed. Note the flattened surface cells which account for the fiber cells often seen in smears. H. and E. ×64.

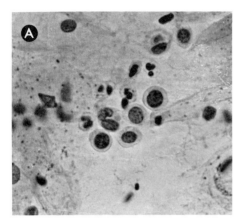
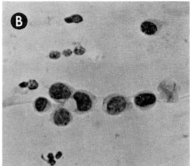
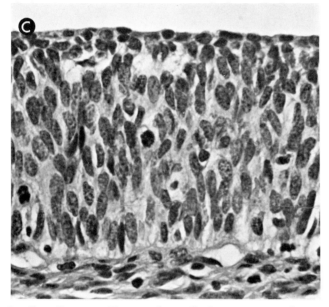

Fig. 10-10. – Small malignant cells. **A** and **B**, cells from a smear of a patient with CIS. Their small size is evident when compared with the other cell types more characteristic of CIS (see Figs. 10-2D, 10-3A, 10-4A, 10-5A, 10-6A, 10-7A and B, 10-8A and B, 10-9A). Such small cells are round to oval in shape; constituent nuclei are of similar configuration. Nuclei have coarsely clumped chromatin and, at times, nucleoli. They may appear in loose groupings, but are rarely syncytial. **C**, histologic section of the same patient whose cytology is shown in **A** and **B**. This section was taken at ×160; other sections in this chapter, except for Figure 10-8D, are ×64. Thus, the small size of the cells constituting this lesion can be readily appreciated.

lar origin, they characteristically appear in clusters. These cells represent about 5% of the malignant population from cases of in situ cancer and only rarely do they predominate.[25]

KERATINIZING CANCER CELL. — These cells are large and irregularly shaped (Fig. 10-9) with an angulate cell outline, at least in some areas. The cytoplasm is characteristically eosinophilic to orangeophilic. The nucleus is ordinarily irregular and markedly hyperchromic, often containing chromatin in large clumps. This contrasts with the vesicular pattern of nuclei in dysplastic cells. These cells occur either singly, in clusters or, at times, in a true syncytial pattern. Keratinizing cancer cells predominate (almost 50% of the cell population) in 40% of the cases in women aged 50 or over. Less than 10% of cells from younger women belong to this category, where they rarely predominate.[29]

SMALL MALIGNANT CELL. — These small cells vary from round or oval to those demonstrating spindling. The nucleus generally occupies a greater proportion of the total cell area (Fig. 10-10) than the previously described types. The nuclear chromatin pattern is coarsely granular or "India ink." Nucleoli are seen at times but not as commonly as their cell counterpart in invasive squamous cancer. The scant cytoplasm is generally pale blue, light green or colorless; uncommonly, it is eosinophilic. These cells represent less than 5% of malignant cells and, like large nonkeratinizing cells, only rarely are they a predominating cell type.

FIBER CELLS. — These cells are long and spindly, being many times longer than their width (Fig. 10-11). The malignant-appearing granular nucleus is almost central to the long axis of the cell. When related to cell diameter, the nucleus is central or slightly eccentric. The portion of the cell in the area of the nucleus may appear to be slightly protuberant. The cytoplasm is usually eosinophilic. They represent less than 3% of the malignant cell population and are only rarely a predominating cell type. These cells are formed due to pressure effects (p. 90) and are ordinarily confined to several layers on the luminal surface of the epithelium.

UNDIFFERENTIATED CANCER CELLS. — These cells, shown in Figure 10-12, conform to the description given for undifferentiated cancer cells on page 114. They may represent about 5% of the malignant population in older women and only rarely predominate. They are the rarest cell type in women under 50 years of age and do not ordinarily manifest themselves as the predominating type.

TADPOLE CELLS. — These cells are elongate with a hyperchromatic bulging nucleus at one end. Cytoplasm is usually eosinophilic. They are only rarely seen in smears from in situ cancer.

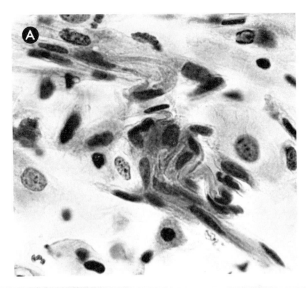

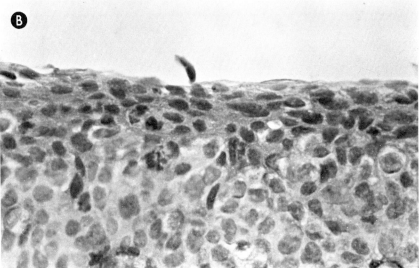

Fig. 10-11.—Fiber cells. **A**, malignant fiber cells in a smear from a patient with CIS of the cervix. When these cells are encountered in smears from intraepithelial neoplasia, they are most commonly found in association with malignant cell types that are either keratinizing or parabasal. Elongate cells, however, are more commonly seen in smears from patients with invasive squamous cancer. **B**, histologic section from the same patient showing the origin of fiber cells. Surface cells are flattened and spindled, although there are parabasal type cells in deeper layers. The surface alteration probably resulted from two forces: luminal pressure in the endocervical canal and growth from the neoplasm below. H. and E. ×160.

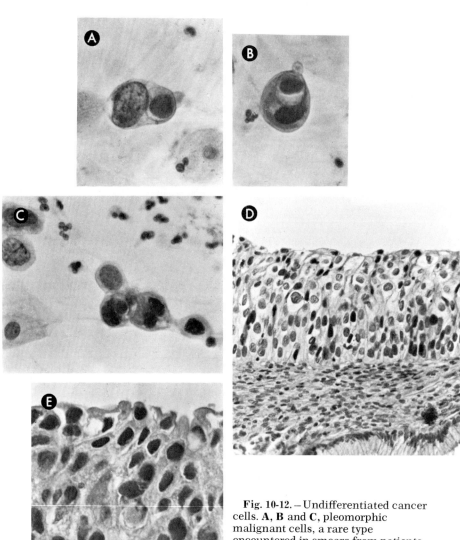

Fig. 10-12. – Undifferentiated cancer cells. **A, B** and **C**, pleomorphic malignant cells, a rare type encountered in smears from patients with CIS, which show variation in size and shape as do constituent nuclei. Nuclei may be in syncytia, chromatin is coarse and nucleoli are often present. This type of cell is more commonly encountered in older patients with CIS. **D** and **E**, histologic sections from the same case as **A, B** and **C**. Irregularity of component cells and nuclei is apparent. H. and E. **A** ×64, **B** ×160.

Cytologic Characteristics of Associated Non-neoplastic Elements

INFLAMMATION

A cervix that has not been subject to exogenous inflammatory stimulus is rarely involved by malignant squamous neoplasia, as evidenced by Ganyon's study of nuns. The greater number of susceptibles for that disease is among a low socioeconomic population in which, unfortunately, chronic cervical inflammatory disease abounds. At least two thirds of patients with in situ cancer will have a significant number of inflammatory cells, usually in the form of degenerated or preserved polymorphonuclear leukocytes. It has been suggested that leukocytic clustering indicates glandular extension of carcinoma in situ.[25] Lymphocytes are only infrequently seen. Unfortunately, the inflammatory response alone offers little diagnostic clue to the underlying process as it often parallels that noted in a routine, nonmalignant hospital and clinic population.

The gross appearance of the cervix usually parallels cytologic inflammatory response. Those patients show erosion, chronic cervicitis or, on occasion, a white plaque. Not unexpectedly, patients over 50 years of age may have a clean-appearing cervix as the portio is completely covered by atrophic squamous epithelium, the squamocolumnar junction appearing high in the endocervical canal. This contrasts with younger women, who often have that junction on the portio. It is worthwhile to reiterate that there is no characteristic gross lesion of in situ cancer of the cervix as that lesion is basically "invisible."

BACTERIAL FLORA

The bacterial flora of carcinoma in situ is commonly abnormal, showing short rods or cocci in at least 75% of cases. The rods and cocci may appear individually or as a mixed flora (Fig. 10-13). In general, more

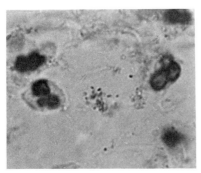

Fig. 10-13. – Papincolaou smear from a patient with CIS showing numerous cocci. Abnormal bacterial flora and polymorphonuclear leukocytes are seen in smears from a majority of patients with CIS. Such findings are nonspecific however, and are of little diagnostic value. Papanicolaou stain, ×500.

rods than cocci will be seen. In up to 30% of cases, Döderlein bacilli may be present[30]; the bacterial flora in these cases is healthy.[29] It is obvious that the bacterial flora is so variable in carcinoma in situ that its diagnostic value is essentially nonexistent.

ERYTHROCYTES

Erythrocytes are usually absent in vaginal fornix smears from patients with carcinoma in situ. However, when material is obtained by scraping the cervix, red blood cells not uncommonly appear in smears.[15, 25] Their presence is probably proportionate to the magnitude of trauma when the smear is taken (Fig. 10-14), which may be influenced by the degree of cervical infection.[27] A few or, occasionally, a moderate number of erythrocytes are encountered. They are more often preserved than degenerated,[30] although such an estimation is difficult as routine Papanicolaou fixation and staining often creates serious artifacts in them. Numerous degenerated erythrocytes are a feature of most cases of invasive cancer.[29, 30]

Fig. 10-14. – Histologic section of the cervix of a patient with carcinoma in situ showing intraepithelial capillaries. This section is from the same patient as shown in Figure 10-7C, but the magnification is greater. By scraping the cervix, vascular spaces may be forcibly disrupted, thus accounting for the presence of erythrocytes in patients with CIS. H. and E. ×160.

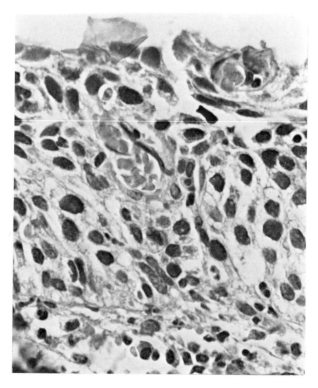

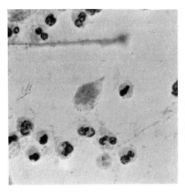

Fig. 10-15.—*Trichomas vaginalis* in a smear from a patient with CIS of the cervix. This organism is frequently encountered in smears from noncancerous patients in a charity clinic population, so that its identification serves no useful purpose in the diagnosis of in situ cancer.

TRICHOMONADS

Trichomonas vaginalis is encountered in smears in about one third of all patients with carcinoma in situ (Fig. 10-15).[10, 14, 26] The parasite may be even more commonly encountered in patients with only inflammatory cervical lesions but by contrast is less common among women who have no cervical disease.[14] An etiological relationship to intraepithelial cancer is tenuous. Assessment of the role of *Trichomonas vaginalis* is complicated by apparent antigenic differences among various strains.[5]

NECROSIS

A necrotic or "dirty" background is usually absent in carcinoma in situ but is mostly present in invasive cancer.[1, 6, 7, 13, 29] Evaluation of a series of smears from patients with in situ cancer revealed that a necrotic background was rare among younger patients. In contrast, around 70% of women over 50 years of age with that lesion had a background composed of degenerated cellular debris (Fig. 10-16). A possible explanation may be that exfoliated normal or neoplastic cells undergo autol-

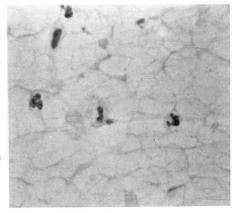

Fig. 10-16.—Smear from an older patient with CIS. The background of this smear forms a mosaic pattern, probably due to the drying of proteinaceous secretions from the vaginal vault. Because secretions remain in the vault for a prolonged period of time in older women, they create an unusual pattern when smears are fixed and stained in the usual manner. The pattern resembles necrosis and may lead to an incorrect cytodiagnosis of invasive cancer.

ysis in the vaginal vault and the resultant debris is not "washed out" by cervical or vaginal secretions as it is likely to be in younger women.

MATURATION INDEX

The maturation index (comparison of the percentage of parabasal, intermediate and superficial cells) of non-neoplastic cells usually reflects expected patterns of maturation for normally menstruating women. Older women with in situ carcinoma have a maturation index that is usually mid or left shifted. They do not ordinarily have an estrogenic pattern. Thus, carcinoma in situ may be seen in a low estrogen environment, as is also common with invasive cervical cancer occurring in the postmenopause. Estrogen may or may not be a necessary ingredient for the *development* of a cervical cancer, but the absence of that hormone does not seem to be a deterrent to its growth. For example, it is possible that intraepithelial neoplasia may have its inception in the postmenopausal period when estrogen levels are significantly depressed. Also, because invasive cervical cancer frequently has its onset in older women, the virtual absence of estrogen at that time is no deterrent to growth and spread of this cancer.

Cellular Patterns in Carcinoma In Situ of the Cervix Uteri

Certain observed cellular patterns can be predictably translated to indicate accurately a subsequent tissue diagnosis in cancer of the cervix. Many investigators have reported correct cytodiagnoses in 80% or more of cases of in situ cancer.[15, 18, 25, 26, 27, 29] Analytical study of the malignant cells also reveals that certain patterns evolve that can be related to specific histopathologic types of intraepithelial cancer. It is germane to subdivide those cell patterns into two groups: those seen in women under the age of 50 and those in women 50 years of age or older. Each of the aforementioned age groups has certain cytologic peculiarities that make such a subdivision of practical value for accurate cytodiagnosis.

CELLULAR PATTERNS IN CARCINOMA IN SITU AMONG WOMEN UNDER THE AGE OF 50 YEARS

Around 80% of women with carcinoma in situ of the uterine cervix will be under the age of 50 years. Therefore, those women comprise the most important population segment when studying that disease. Such patients also have cytologic features allowing for optimal diagnostic predictability of in situ cancer.

Table 10-1 lists the per cent distribution of malignant cells in smears from females under 50 years of age who harbor intraepithelial cancer.

TABLE 10-1.—MALIGNANT CELL DIFFERENTIAL AMONG WOMEN
UNDER THE AGE OF 50 YEARS—PER CENT DISTRIBUTION

CELL TYPE	PER CENT OF TOTAL CELL POPULATION (39 CASES)
1. Parabasal cancer cell	35.4
2. Clustered cancer cell	34.9
3. Keratinizing cancer cell	15.6
4. Large cell, nonkeratinizing	5.3
5. Undifferentiated cancer cell	4.1
6. Small cancer cell	2.6
7. Fiber cell	2.1

It is readily apparent that round or oval, usually isodiametric forms, similar in size to parabasal cells, predominate overwhelmingly. Such an observation has been made repeatedly by numerous workers[3, 4, 15, 18, 25, 26, 29] For example, Reagan and Hamonic[18] found that 85.71% of cells from in situ carcinoma were either round, oval or ellipsoidal, in order of frequency. These findings represent an important standard for the cytodiagnosis of intraepithelial cancer.

Analysis of the predominant malignant cell type in a given case of in situ cancer in a younger woman parallels the per cent distribution, also proving to be of excellent diagnostic value. Table 10-2 shows the predominant malignant cell type per case.

In 30 cases (77%) in this age group parabasal or clustered cancer cells predominated. Of those, 19 cases had a malignant cell population of at least 90% of parabasal or clustered cancer cells, associated with 10% of keratinizing cancer cells in 5 cases or undifferentiated cancer cells in 2 instances. Another 10 smears contained a malignant cell population of 70% to 80% of either malignant parabasal or clustered cancer cells, associated most often with small numbers of keratinizing cancer cells or rarely those of undifferentiated or large, nonkeratinizing types. One case had an equal number of malignant parabasal and fiber cells. Keratinizing cancer cells predominated in 5 cases and they accounted for 50%–100% of the malignant cell population. They were most often associated with parabasal type or clustered cancer cells, although at times fiber or undifferentiated cancer cells accompanied.

TABLE 10-2.—PREDOMINANT MALIGNANT CELL TYPE PER CASE AMONG
WOMEN UNDER THE AGE OF 50 YEARS—39 CASES

CELL TYPE	NUMBER OF CASES	PER CENT
1. Clustered cancer cell	17	43.6 ⎫
2. Parabasal cancer cell	11	28.2 ⎪
3. Clustered cancer and parabasal cancer cells in equal numbers	1	2.6 ⎬ 77
4. Parabasal and fiber cells in equal numbers	1	2.6 ⎭
5. Keratinizing cancer cell	5	12.7
6. Large cell, nonkeratinizing	2	5.1
7. Small cancer cell	1	2.6
8. Undifferentiated cancer cell	1	2.6

Predominating large, nonkeratinizing, small or undifferentiated cancer cells usually accounted for at least 80% of the malignant cell population in those particular cases; if other cell types were present, they were of parabasal type or clustered cancer cell variety.

Thus, whether one utilizes percentage distribution or predominant malignant cell type per case, the cytodiagnosis of in situ cancer in women under 50 years of age is highly predictable. Unfortunately, such findings cannot be translated to smears from older women with in situ cancer of the cervix, as will be evident in the following section.

Cellular Patterns in Carcinoma In Situ Among Women 50 Years of Age or Older

About 20% of women with carcinoma in situ of the cervix will be 50 years of age or older. Table 10-3 lists the per cent distribution of malignant cells in smears from females in that age group. It will be noted that the constituent cell population deviates significantly from that of younger women. More specifically, there is a 2.6 times increase in the number of keratinizing cancer cells. Those of parabasal type and clustered cancer variety are almost one-half as frequent, while undifferentiated cancer cells are more commonly encountered.

An analysis of the predominant malignant cell type per case magnifies the true nature of the discrepancy in cellular patterns between younger and older women with carcinoma in situ of the cervix. Table 10-4 shows that the smears from 95.2% of cases contained either keratinizing, clustered cancer or parabasal type cells as the predominant cell. It is noteworthy that every case in this group had either clustered cancer, parabasal or keratinizing cancer cells in variable numbers. Keratinizing cancer cells were the most common malignant cell in 12 (57.1%) of these cases, whereas the clustered cancer or parabasal type cell predominated in 8 (38.1%). One case (4.8%) had a predominant cell population of undifferentiated cancer cells.

Further analysis of the 12 cases in which keratinizing cancer cells predominated revealed that this cell type accounted for 40% to 90% of

TABLE 10-3.—Malignant Cell Differential
Among Women 50 Years of Age or Older—
Per Cent Distribution

Cell Type	Per Cent of Total Cell Population (21 Cases)
1. Keratinizing cancer cell	41.5
2. Clustered cancer cell	21.4 ⎫
	⎬ 41.4
3. Parabasal cancer cell	20.0 ⎭
4. Undifferentiated cancer cell	13.3
5. Large cell, nonkeratinizing	2.8
6. Fiber cell	1.0

TABLE 10-4.—PREDOMINANT MALIGNANT CELL TYPE PER CASE AMONG
WOMEN 50 YEARS OF AGE OR OLDER—21 CASES

CELL TYPE	NUMBER OF CASES	PER CENT
1. Keratinizing cancer cell	12	57.1
2. Clustered cancer cell	5	
3. Parabasal cancer cell	2	38.1
4. Parabasal and clustered cancer cells in equal numbers	1	
5. Undifferentiated cancer cell	1	4.8

the total cell population. Nine of those 12 cases were complemented by
10%–40% of malignant parabasal cells; in 3 cases, parabasal and clustered cancer cells were the only associated cells (10%–40%). In 3 other
cases, parabasal or clustered cancer cells were combined with 20%–
30% of undifferentiated cancer cells; in another 2, large nonkeratinizing cancer cells were present at 30% each; and, in 1 other, there were
10% fiber cells. In each of 2 cases, keratinizing cancer cells and undifferentiated cells were present in equal numbers (40% each), complemented by 20% of parabasal-type cells.

In the 8 smears in which parabasals predominated, they accounted
for 60% to 100% of the total cell population. In 5 of the 8, keratinizing
cancer cells were associated, comprising from 10%–40% of the total
cell population; in 2 of the 5, there were also 10% of undifferentiated
cancer cells. In 1 case, a cell population of 90% clustered cancer cells
was combined with 10% of undifferentiated cancer cells.

In the 1 case with a predominating cell type other than parabasal or
keratinizing cancer cell, 70% were undifferentiated, 20% keratinizing
and 10% parabasal-type malignant cells.

SALIENT COMPARATIVE FEATURES OF CELLULAR PATTERNS AMONG YOUNGER AND OLDER PATIENTS WITH CARCINOMA IN SITU OF THE CERVIX

The cytologic picture in the aged can be characterized best by the
great number of keratinizing cancer cells mixed with a lesser number
of parabasal-type cells. That contrasts with the almost constant prepon-
derance of parabasals or clustered cancer cells in younger women. In
contradistinction to smears from younger women, those from older
women often had a "dirty" background, in common with invasive
smears, probably related to a deficiency of secretions to wash out exfoliated and degenerated cells. Older women had a maturation index characterized by a left shift, comparable to that expected for their advanced
age. The younger women reflected maturation indices paralleling that
expected for active menstruation. Inflammatory cells, bacterial flora,
erythrocytes and trichomonads were not significant differential features.

What is the explanation for the divergent malignant cell populations among the two age groups? In younger females, it is logical to assume that the isodiametric, fairly small, round cells originate as a consequence of active replication from basal, parabasal or reserve (prosoplastic) cells.[7] The just-noted cellular elements have features of similar size and shape, notwithstanding fine morphologic differences. Cell replication in these women ordinarily proceeds along orderly lines, influenced in part by the normal hormone milieu of the younger women. In that context, it is of interest that Krieg and Reagan found that induced cervical cancer in noncastrated mice progressed to invasion more slowly than in castrates.[11] Eventually, invasion may take place in the human; the lesion may remain static or undergo transformation to different cell types of in situ carcinoma or, possibly, regress. In situ patterns seen in older women with predominant keratinizing or even more undifferentiated cells probably originate from patterns established at an earlier age. For example, older women have certain cell types unusual for those of in situ cancer in younger women, but there is a close association with parabasal type cells, common to the latter age group. The presence of parabasal-type cells in older women possibly represents an ancestral holdover from an earlier age. The newer, more undifferentiated cell types in older women may indicate either that a particular clone of cells is gaining ascendency or that there is a modification of pre-existent cells due to a change in hormonal status, i.e., estrogen deficiency. Assuming that in situ cancer may eventually become invasive, a change in cell patterns would be logically anticipated, as cell types of invasive cancer are usually radically different from most in situ lesions. However, cell types of invasive cancer bear a much greater similarity to patterns observed in older than in younger females with carcinoma in situ. It is convenient to postulate that cells from in situ lesions in the aged, rather than from younger women, have a greater potentiality to become aggressive, as invasive cervical malignancy is also more common with advancing age. Development of invasive cervical malignancy in younger females is not dependent on a change in hormonal status but is related primarily to biologic activity of the neoplastic cells. Keratinizing tendencies of some cells may be related more to vitality than to biologic senescence.[16]

Cytologic Findings in Developmental Carcinoma In Situ of the Cervix

In 1962, Reagan and associates[23] described the earliest, or developmental, stages of carcinoma in situ of the cervix. The lesion was considered to arise from metaplastic reserve cells. Such elements were comparable in size to cells of reserve origin but were larger than those of carcinoma in situ. Constituent cells were more often isolated and in sheets than cells of in situ cancer but were less commonly in syncytia. In these respects, they bore closer similarity to cell arrangements in dysplasia. The number of round or oval cell shapes was intermediate between those observed in dysplasia and carcinoma in situ, being 63%. Cells of the developmental lesion were more often eosinophilic than cells of dysplasia or carcinoma in situ; conversely, cytoplasmic basophilia was less common than either of the aforementioned. Nuclear diameters of developmental carcinoma in situ were small, being less than those of dysplasia or in situ cancer. The finely granular nuclear chromatin pattern was similar to dysplastic cells, while coarse granularity was not nearly as common as in cells of in situ carcinoma. Chromocenters were much commoner than in cells of in situ cancer and in that regard were comparable to those of reserve cells. Cytoplasmic vacuolization corresponded more so to reserve cells of ordinary carcinoma in situ. According to the foregoing parameters, the constituent cells of developmental carcinoma in situ seem to possess characteristics intermediate between cells of dysplasia and carcinoma in situ. Their greatest similarity is to reserve (or prosoplastic) cells, from which they undoubtedly originate.

Koss and Durfee[9] described some cellular changes similar to those just noted in cytologic smears taken from 29 to 71 months prior to the development of carcinoma in situ. Their 4 patients averaged 34 years, whereas the 30 women in the Reagan *et al.* series averaged 36.33 years.

Correlated Cytohistologic Patterns Observed in Carcinoma In Situ of the Cervix

A histologic diagnosis of carcinoma in situ is established by the following criteria:

1. The "basement membrane"* of the surface or contiguous glands (or crypts) has not been breeched by the epithelial abnormality.

2. There must be a definite loss in polarity of cells from the basal layer to the luminal border of the epithelium. Because of surrounding pressure effects, from the cells below and the lumen of the cervical canal above, the top few cell layers may be parallel to the general plane of the parent tissue, i.e., parallel to the plane of the endocervical canal. Nevertheless, the top cell layers still must show abnormal nuclear characteristics.

3. The individual cells must show malignant nuclei with altered nuclear-cytoplasmic ratios. Anaplasia is the most important single characteristic of carcinoma in situ of the cervix.[17]

---

*Electron microscopic studies have demonstrated that in the cervix uteri there is no true basement membrane as is common of many epithelia of the body. Instead, it is composed of dense stroma.

4. Mitotic figures are of substantive value only when found in the upper half of the epithelial thickness and may be seen in the metaphase or as "pathologic" types. It will be remembered that mitotic figures are normally observed in the germinative layer and, on occasion, in parabasal cells.

The general principles of the above description must be applied to the diagnosis of carcinoma in situ; however, the individual anaplastic cells (part 3) may vary greatly in their morphology. Siegler[26] described five histologic, and correlating cytologic, types of in situ cancer of the cervix. His types can be more conveniently modified into four histologic varieties which demonstrate excellent cytologic correlation. They are as follows:

Varieties of Histologic Patterns Constituting In Situ Cancer (With Cytologic Correlation)

I. PARABASAL CELL TYPE. — This is the commonest pattern. The constituent cells are regular in size, round to oval, and mimic those of parabasal or reserve (prosoplastic) layers of the cervical squamous epithelium (Fig. 10-17, *A*).

Cytologic preparations from such cases usually reveal cells of parabasal type, clustered cancer cells or large cell, nonkeratinizing elements. Developmental carcinoma in situ may be associated with such a

Fig. 10-17. — Parabasal cell type. **A**, histologic section showing the parabasal type of CIS. There is maintenance of an isodiametric, round-to-oval type throughout the epithelial thickness and a mitotic figure appears about six cells beneath the surface. This histologic pattern is usually associated with smears containing parabasal cancer cells. However, large nonkeratinizing cancer cells may be associated with an almost indistinguishable histologic pattern. H. and E. ×160. **B**, an isolated parabasal cell (*center*) in a smear from the same patient as shown in **A**.

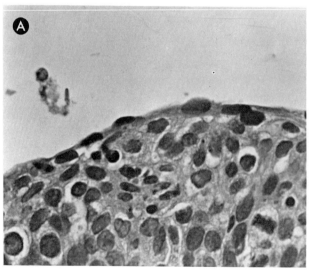
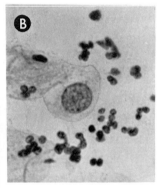

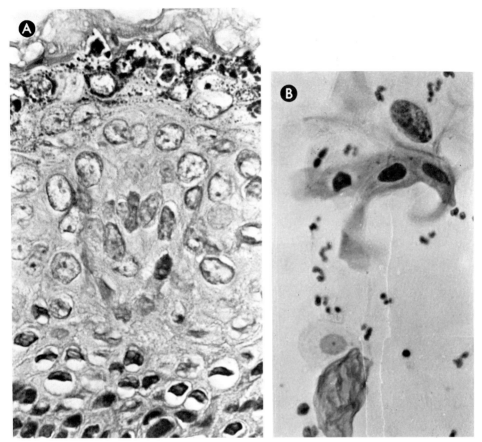

Fig. 10-18. – Keratinizing cell type. **A,** histologic section of the keratinizing type of CIS. A keratin layer is at the top of the figure with a row of cells containing keratohyalin granules below. Observe that cells with altered nuclear/cytoplasmic ratios extend throughout the entire epithelial thickness. H. and E. ×160. **B,** cells characteristically seen in smears from patients with the keratinizing variety of CIS of the cervix. They are almost always irregular with eosinophilic cytoplasm and irregular nuclei with a coarsely clumped chromatin pattern. Note the anucleate squamous cell.

histologic picture. Constituent cells may differ in size from one case to another, primarily a reflection of the cell of origin (Fig. 10-17, *B*).

II. KERATINIZING CELL TYPE. – This is an unusual pattern in younger individuals but is very common in older women. At times a variant of this lesion is seen in developmental carcinoma in situ. The histologic pattern consists of a disorderly maturation of abnormal keratinizing elements, generally arranged in a haphazard pattern. There may be associated leukoplakia in about one third of cases. Often, lower areas of the epithelium contain isodiametric round cells. This suggests that the more superficial layers may represent dedifferentiation of more differentiated, deeper occurring cells. The cytoplasm, especially in cells from the upper one half of the epithelial thickness, is fairly abundant and is keratinized (Fig. 10-18, *A*).

The cytologic pattern is usually predominantly composed of keratinizing cancer cells, although commonly a variable number of parabasal type are present (Fig. 10-18, *B*).

III. PLEOMORPHIC CELL TYPE.—This is a rare pattern, a reflection of the seldom occurrence of pleomorphic cells in carcinoma in situ. Such a histologic pattern will usually be noted in older women. The constituent elements are arranged in a haphazard fashion and are composed of irregular cells of various sizes, both in regard to nuclei and cytoplasm. The cytoplasm is not keratinized (Fig. 10-19, *A*).

Figs. 10-19.—Pleomorphic cell type. **A,** histologic section from the surface of a pleomorphic variety of CIS. Cell irregularity is obvious. There is a mitotic figure a few cells below the surface. H. and E. ×160. **B,** a smear from the same case as **A.** Two malignant cells are shown which vary markedly in size and shape. They have a cyanophilic cytoplasm and the variation in the size and shape of the nucleus is apparent.

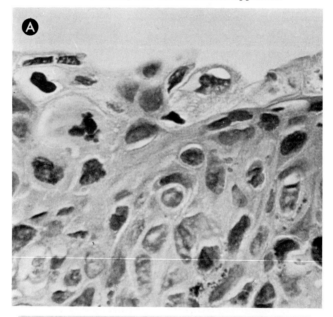

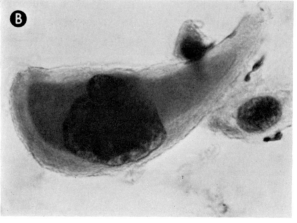

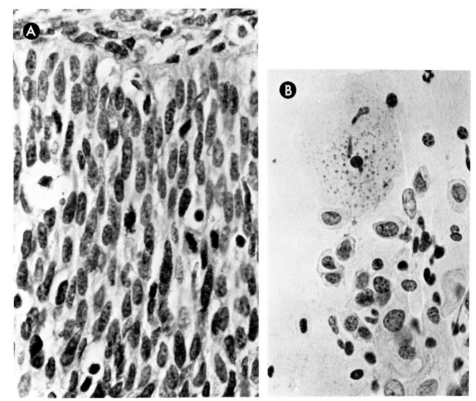

Fig. 10-20.—Small cell type. **A,** histologic section of a type of CIS composed of small malignant cells which show similar characteristics throughout the entire epithelial thickness. H. and E. ×160. **B,** a smear from the same case as **A.** Very small cancer cells are seen with difficulty. Their size contrasts sharply with the normal superficial cell at the top of the figure.

The cytology smear, with its complement of undifferentiated cells, more closely resembles an invasive lesion rather than one that is actually in situ. Ancillary background features such as blood and necrotic debris may be very helpful in arriving at a correct cytodiagnosis; i.e., more blood and necrotic debris will be observed in invasive lesions (Fig. 10-19, *B*).

IV. SMALL CELL TYPE.—Once again, this is an unusual histologic or cytologic pattern. Tissue sections demonstrate regularity of constituent cells similar to the parabasal (type I) histologic pattern. However, close inspection usually shows that the cells are quite small, very similar in size to those of the basal cell layer. Some nuclear irregularities are detectable under high magnification (Fig. 10-20, *A*).

The cytology is as described for the small malignant cell. It is pertinent that such a cell type occurs more commonly with invasive cancers. As with the pleomorphic type (type III), background features may have to be relied upon for a correct cytodiagnosis, i.e., in situ vs. invasion (Fig. 10-20, *B*).

In general, the predominating malignant cells seen on smear study correlate well with histologic findings.

Practical Diagnostic Features for the Cytologic Diagnosis of Carcinoma In Situ of the Cervix

As indicated in a preceding section, it is necessary that all cytology slides be meticulously screened and appropriately dotted by an experienced observer. Slide analysis commences by examining cells indicated by dots which should represent the most dedifferentiated elements. Then the entire slide should be scanned to determine the number of significantly altered cells. Associated features, such as normal cells, inflammation, Trichomonas, necrosis, blood, etc., should be assessed. If it is decided that the most atypical cells represent probable neoplasm, it is profitable to attempt to determine whether it is possible to trace transitional forms from benign to malignant. Such transitions are usually easier to follow in lesions up to and including in situ cancer. A hiatus from benign to frankly malignant cells is more common with invasive cancer. Background features are only modifiers. For example, *severe* necrosis, while common in invasive cancer, is rarely noted with in situ lesions. However, moderate degrees of necrosis may be seen in either invasive or in situ malignancy, in the latter primarily in older women. A definitive diagnosis in the presence of only a few severely altered cells is dangerous and ordinarily indicates the need for immediate repeat fractionated specimens, i.e., vaginal pool, cervical scrape, endocervical or, at times, endometrial aspiration. Thus, while cytodiagnosis is primarily based on individual cell changes, the cell distribution (cancer trend) indicates commonly accurate prediction of subsequent tissue findings.

REFERENCES

1. Campos, J. R. de C.: Symposium on carcinoma in situ, Acta cytol. 5:439, 1961.
2. Foraker, A. G.: An analysis of nuclear size and nuclear:cytoplasmic ratio in the histological diagnosis of intraepithelial carcinoma of the cervix uteri, Cancer 7:884, 1954.
3. Graham, R. M.: Symposium on carcinoma in situ, Acta cytol. 5:425, 1961.
4. Graham, R. M.: *The Cytologic Diagnosis of Cancer* (2d ed.; Philadelphia: W. B. Saunders Company, 1963).
5. Honigberg, B. M.: Pathogenicity of fresh isolates of Trichomonas vaginalis: "the mouse assay" versus clinical and pathologic findings, Acta cytol. 10:353, 1966.
6. Jenny, J., and Wacek, A.: Symposium on carcinoma in situ, Acta cytol. 5:446, 1961.
7. Johnson, L. D., *et al.*: The histogenesis of carcinoma in situ of the uterine cervix, Cancer 17:213, 1964.
8. Johnston, D. G.: Cytoplasmic:nuclear ratios in the cytological diagnosis of cancer, Cancer 5:945, 1952.
9. Koss, L. G., and Durfee, G. L.: Cytological changes preceding the appearance of in situ carcinoma of the uterine cervix, Cancer 8:295, 1955.
10. Koss, L. G., and Wolinska, W. H.: Trichomonas vaginalis cervicitis and its relationship to cervical cancer, Cancer 12:1171, 1959.
11. Krieg, A. F., and Reagan, J. W.: Carcinogenesis of the cervix uteri in castrate mice, Lab. Invest. 10:581, 1961.
12. Lindner, A.: Suggested explanation for accuracy of the Papanicolaou method for cytologic diagnosis, Am. J. Clin. Path. 29:43, 1958.

13. Montalvo-Ruiz, L.: Symposium on carcinoma in situ, Acta cytol. 5:447, 1961.
14. Naguib, S. M., *et al.*: Epidemiologic study of trichomoniasis in normal women, Obst. & Gynec. 27:607, 1966.
15. Okagaki, T., *et al.*: Diagnosis of anaplasia and carcinoma in situ by differential cell counts, Acta cytol. 6:343, 1962.
16. Old, J. W., *et al.*: Squamous carcinoma in situ of the uterine cervix, Cancer 18:1598, 1965.
17. Reagan, J. W.: Carcinoma in Situ, in Wartman, W. B. (ed.): *Year Book of Pathology and Clinical Pathology* (Chicago: Year Book Medical Publishers, 1955).
18. Reagan, J. W., and Hamonic, M. J.: The cellular pathology in carcinoma in situ, Cancer 9:385, 1959.
19. Reagan, J. W., and Moore, R. D.: Morphology of the malignant squamous cell, Am. J. Path. 28:105, 1952.
20. Reagan, J. W., and Ng, A. B. P.: *The Cells of Uterine Adenocarcinoma* (Baltimore: Williams & Wilkins Company, 1965).
21. Reagan, J. W., and Patten, S. F.: Analytic study of cellular changes in carcinoma in situ, squamous cell cancer, and adenocarcinoma of uterine cervix, Clin. Obst. & Gynec. 4:1097, 1961.
22. Reagan, J. W., *et al.*: Analytical study of the cells in cervical squamous cancer, Lab. Invest. 6:241, 1957.
23. Reagan, J. W., *et al.*: Developmental stages of in situ carcinoma in uterine cervix: an analytical study of the cells, Acta cytol. 6:538, 1962.
24. Richart, R. M., and Wilbanks, G. D.: The chromosomes of human intraepithelial neoplasia: report of 14 cases of cervical intraepithelial neoplasia and review, Cancer Res. 26:60, 1966.
25. Roberts, T. W., and Linkins, T.: Differentiation between intramucosal and invasive carcinoma of the cervix by cytologic smear. Is it reliable? Acta cytol. 8:280, 1964.
26. Siegler, E. E.: Symposium on carcinoma in situ, Acta cytol. 5:428, 1961.
27. Turnbull, L. A.: Symposium on carcinoma in situ, Acta cytol. 5:448, 1961.
28. Wakonig-Vaartaja, R., and Kirkland, J. A.: A correlated chromosomal and histopathologic study of pre-invasive lesions of the cervix, Cancer 18:1101, 1965.
29. Wied, G. L.: The potentialities of the smear technique for the differentiation of noninvasive and invasive cervical carcinoma, Am. J. Obst. & Gynec. 71:793, 1956.
30. Wied, G. L., *et al.*: Cytology of invasive cervical carcinoma and carcinoma in situ, Ann. New York Acad. Sc. 97:759, 1962.

CHAPTER 11

The Cytopathology of Invasive Squamous Carcinoma of the Cervix

Introduction and Definition

AN INVASIVE SQUAMOUS cell carcinoma of the cervix is one that has penetrated beyond the confines of the "basement membrane." For practical purposes, microinvasive cancer (tumors 0.5 cm. or less in depth of penetration) is excluded from the preceding definition, because it displays biologic behavior of a distinctly different nature. For example, even though vascular invasion may be noted in microinvasive cancer, metastasis is nonetheless rare. This contrasts with cancers presenting deeper penetration, as cancer confined to the cervix on clinical examination affects regional lymph nodes in 20% of instances.

Cervical cancer is customarily classified in four clinical stages. The stages correlate tumor extent and prognosis; greater spread is associated with a progressively poorer outlook. Stage I cancer is confined to the cervix; stage II extends beyond the cervix but does not involve the lateral pelvic wall or the lower one third of the vagina. Stage III involves either the lateral pelvic wall or the lower one third of the vagina; stage IV cancers show greater extension than those of stage III with involvement of the urinary bladder, rectal wall or other more distant spread. The preceding stages of cancer are invariably symptomatic and when diagnosed manifest a visible cervical lesion. Accordingly, the method of choice in initial diagnostic study should be a tissue biopsy. Since the paramount role of cytology is to discover invisible lesions, cytodiagnosis plays a purely secondary role in the diagnosis of invasive (visible) cancer. Additionally, smears from patients with invasive cancer may be negative in up to 5% of cases. Necrosis, blood and inflammation may be so prominent in such smears that tumor cells are either not present or are obscured by debris. Despite the shortcomings of cytodiagnosis in such cases, we recommend a routine cervicovaginal smear. The clinician may conceivably underestimate the condition of the cervix harboring invasive cancer, or biopsy the wrong area; in such instances, biopsy might be negative while a smear is positive. The prevalence of such circumstances warrants substantial attention to proper recognition of malignant cells from invasive cervical cancer.

Clinical Features

The patient with invasive cervical squamous cancer might be characterized as follows: she is in her middle or late forties, from a poor socioeconomic background and has had many pregnancies. Careful history reveals either marriage or coitus commencing at an early age. A positive history for syphilis or pelvic inflammatory disease might be obtained. It is unlikely that she is either Jewish or a Catholic nun.[17] The reader is directed to an excellent and amusing one page article by Rappolt[12] describing many facets of the prototype with cervical cancer.

Her presenting complaints are usually abnormal vaginal bleeding and/or discharge. Other symptoms such as pain, sensation of a tumor mass, etc., ordinarily indicate advanced disease.

The physician identifies a lesion of the cervix of variable size that is either ulcerated or, less commonly, exophytic. Visual inspection, bimanual examination or biopsy further categorizes the neoplasm into one of the international stages of tumor extension.

Cytologic Characteristics of Associated Non-neoplastic Elements

INFLAMMATION. – Invasive cancer is more commonly accompanied by large numbers of inflammatory cells than either dysplasia or carcinoma in situ. Polymorphonuclear leukocytes in varying stages of degeneration are the cells usually encountered. However, smears from an exophytic tumor may contain only neoplastic cells. Should the necrotic base of a lesion be sampled, smears may only show necrotic debris in which there are scattered segmented neutrophils, often degenerated.[7, 13, 15, 20]

BACTERIAL FLORA. – In contrast with smears from carcinoma in situ, those from invasive cancer are more prone to contain secondary bacterial invaders, usually gram-positive cocci,[6] occasionally accompanied by gram-negative rods. Such flora may be masked by attendant debris. It is most unusual to have a normal flora of Döderlein bacilli with invasive cancer.[6, 10, 20, 21]

ERYTHROCYTES. – Over 90% of smears from invasive squamous cancer contain significant numbers of erythrocytes,[21] the majority evidencing some degeneration.[15, 21] By contrast, only about one third of the smears from in situ cancer reveal red blood cells characteristically in

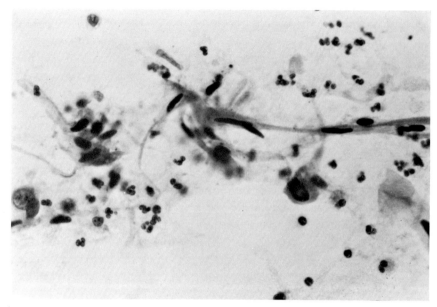

Fig. 11-1.—Smear from invasive cancer. The cytoplasm of these malignant cells is eosinophilic and the shape varies from those that are fiberlike to those that are small and irregular. Many of the smaller cells have irregular, hyperchromatic nuclei occupying a larger percentage of the total cell area than is usual in cells of carcinoma in situ.

small numbers and well preserved. That finding in carcinoma in situ is commonly due to the trauma incident to taking the smear from a lesion with superficially located capillaries.

TRICHOMONADS.—Prevalence of *Trichomonas vaginalis* in smears from invasive cancer has been variously noted to be less or more common than in smears from in situ cancer.[8, 9, 21] The organism may be obscured by the presence of much blood and debris in certain advanced cases.

NECROSIS.—Smears from invasive cancer commonly have a background composed of amorphous debris, derived from the necrotic tissue of degenerated tumor.[7, 15] The number of cases containing necrotic debris, as well as their magnitude, is dependent on the amount of tumor necrosis and the area from which the smear is taken (Fig. 11-1). It is unusual to observe smears showing a "dirty" or necrotic background from patients with in situ cancer, except in older women.[4]

MATURATION INDEX.—The maturation index from patients with invasive cancer parallels that expected for their age and menstrual status.

Number of Malignant Cells and the Cancer Trend

Smears from invasive cancer either contain an overwhelming number of frankly malignant cells or such elements may be uncommon due to dilution by blood and/or debris.[11, 13] The number of malignant cells observed is related in part to the location from which the smear is taken.[21] The hiatus between normal and malignant cells may be extreme when a minimal dysplastic or in situ component exists, contrasting sharply with smear findings from the in situ lesion.[19, 20] However, small invasive lesions with accompanying in situ cancer may reveal a gradual blend from normal to frankly malignant cells.

The Malignant Cells of Invasive Squamous Cancer

As indicated, smears from patients with invasive cancer may contain a wide spectrum of neoplastic cells, sometimes similar to those seen in dysplasia or carcinoma in situ, but more commonly characteristic of invasive cancer. Thus, cytosmear differentiation between carcinoma in situ and invasive cancer in the main utilizes cellular features of a qualitative nature. Cells from invasive cancer are often grouped as syncytial masses; individual cells are usually smaller with a more irregular nucleus and cytoplasm than those of in situ cancer. Cytoplasm of cells from invasive cancer varies from eosinophilic (in instances of the common keratinizing cancer) to cyanophilic or indeterminate, whereas in carcinoma in situ cytoplasmic basophilia greatly predominates. Nuclei of invasive cancer cells are smaller than those of carcinoma in situ but nevertheless occupy a greater proportion of the cellular area (Fig. 11-1). Nuclear chromatin of cells from invasive cancer varies from

Fig. 11-2.—Malignant cells of invasive squamous cell cancer. **A,** cells from a smear of a patient with large-cell, nonkeratinizing squamous cell cancer of the cervix which have prominent nucleoli and a finely dispersed nuclear chromatin pattern. Cells of this type of cancer are usually more regular than cells of the keratinizing variety. **B,** histologic section from the same patient whose cells are depicted in **A.** Notice the regular, generally oval-shaped cells and nuclei, the prominent nucleoli and absence of keratinization.

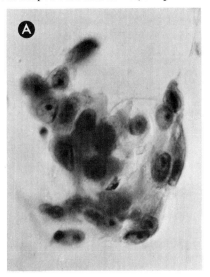
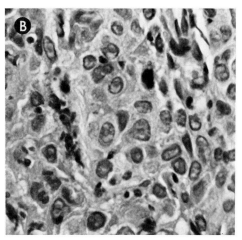

TABLE 11-1.–INVASIVE SQUAMOUS CANCER OF THE
CERVIX – MALIGNANT CELL DIFFERENTIAL – %DISTRIBUTION

CELL TYPE	PER CENT DISTRIBUTION
Undifferentiated cancer cell	30.0
Keratinizing cancer cell	23.5
Small cancer cell	21.6
Large cell, nonkeratinizing	13.3
Parabasal cancer cell	6.5
Fiber cells	5.1

finely granular to opaque, with most of the cells more heavily granulated than those most commonly seen in carcinoma in situ (Fig. 11-1). Nucleoli are far more common in cells from invasive cancer than in those encountered in carcinoma in situ. Macronucleoli are a feature of invasive cancer and are not usually seen in smears from in situ cancer (Fig. 11-2).[13, 14]

Specific cell types encountered in smears from invasive cancer, and their relative prevalence, are indicated in Table 11-1. The majority of cells present in smears from invasive squamous cancer can be conveniently subdivided into three major varieties[14]: nonkeratinizing (including both cells that are undifferentiated and large, nonkeratinizing cells), keratinizing (including keratinizing cancer and fiber cells) and small malignant cells. In a given case, there may be sufficient variation in cell pattern so that there are representatives of more than one major variety. Pertinent features of the three major cell varieties are specified in Table 11-2.

The following general remarks, referable to each cell type, are for assistance in recognition and differentiation.

TABLE 11-2.–CYTOLOGIC FEATURES OF THREE MAJOR VARIETIES OF CELLS ENCOUNTERED IN
SQUAMOUS CELL CARCINOMA OF THE UTERINE CERVIX

CELL FEATURE	KERATINIZING	CELL TYPE LARGE CELL, NONKERATINIZING	SMALL CELL
Cell area*	1	2	3
Nuclear area*	2	1	3
Relative nuclear area*	3	2	1
Tadpole and elongate cells	15%	0.4%	0.2%
Syncytial masses	13.5%	23.12%	12.27%
Nuclear features			
Finely granular chromatin	22.12%	20.29%	12.62%
Coarse granular chromatin	58.97%	76.42%	79.53%
Opaque	18.91%	3.34%	7.85%
Nucleoli per case	5.04	23.73	19.91
Free nuclei per case	21.79	122.83	50.71

*1 = largest size; 2 = intermediate size; 3 = smallest size.
From Reagan, J. W., Hamonic, M. J., and Wentz, W. B.: Lab. Invest. 6:241, 1957.

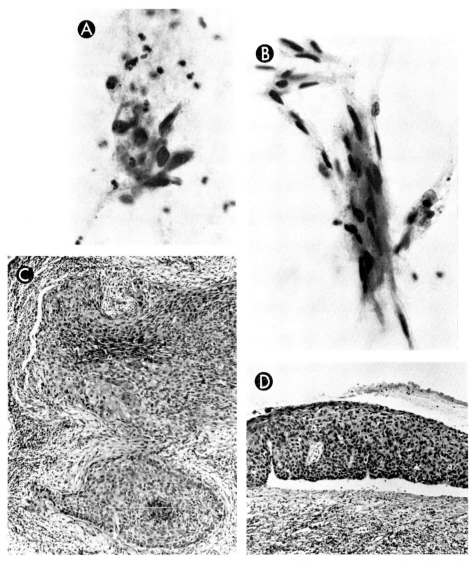

Fig. 11-3. – Keratinizing cells of invasive squamous cell cancer. **A,** irregular cells with eosinophilic cytoplasm in a smear from a patient with keratinizing cancer. Nuclei of variable size and shape are hyperchromatic. **B,** malignant fiber cells such as these are most commonly observed in patients with invasive keratinizing cancer. However, similar cells may also be seen in smears from patients with in situ cancer. **C,** histologic section from a patient with invasive keratinizing cancer. Even at this magnification the variation in cell shape, as seen in **A** and **B,** is readily apparent. **D,** histologic section of an in situ cancer which was adjacent to the invasive malignancy seen in **C.** Note the distinct keratinizing tendencies of the epithelioma – the keratinizing type of in situ cancer. Invasive cancer associated with keratinizing in situ cancer is always of the keratinizing variety.

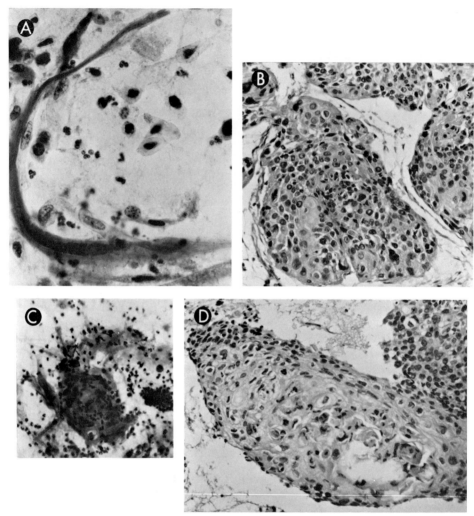

Fig. 11-4. – Keratinizing cells of invasive squamous cell cancer. **A,** an unusually large, malignant fiber cell from the invasive keratinizing cancer shown in **B**. Note that the nucleus does not necessarily displace the cell outline. **B,** histologic section of an invasive keratinizing cancer showing elongation and distortion of cells at the periphery of the growth. **C,** the cell grouping in the center of this smear shows a poorly formed pearl. Such a feature is characteristic of keratinizing cancer as shown in **D**. It is important to keep in mind that pearls of a somewhat different character may also be observed in smears from patients with inflammatory processes and in situ cancer. **D,** histologic section of an invasive keratinizing cancer from the patient in **C**, showing cell distortion and elongation at both the central and peripheral areas. The pearl depicted in **C** could have conceivably come from the hole in the central area of this cell group.

Keratinizing Cancer Cells

This cell type may also be seen in carcinoma in situ, with cellular characteristics resembling those seen in invasive cancer. However, there are certain pertinent differences. For example, cytoplasmic orangeophilia is observed only rarely in keratinizing cells from in situ cancer, where they are usually eosinophilic.

Of all cell types encountered, keratinizing cancer cells have the greatest frequency of opaque nuclei and seldom contain nucleoli. At times, the dense chromatin may represent a degenerative phenomenon, indicating lessened cell viability.

Cell shape and arrangement in smears from cases of keratinizing cancer deserve special mention. In no other neoplasm, save leiomyosarcoma, is it so common to encounter elongated cells.[1] Such neoplastic elements are observed uncommonly when studying material from instances of carcinoma in situ or dysplasia.[2, 3] Elongated squamous cells may also be present in smears from inflammatory conditions, following the trauma of delivery or in postpartum smears.[5, 8, 16] At times, the cells are arranged in tight groups (epithelial pearls), malignant pearls being most commonly associated with invasive cancer.[1] However, cells arranged in a pearl pattern may also be found in inflammatory conditions, dysplasia or, rarely, carcinoma in situ, so that proper identification must rely on precise delineation of nuclear and cytoplasmic characteristics (Figs. 11-3 and 11-4).

Large Nonkeratinizing Cells

These cells often have features resembling those of adenocarcinoma, such as cell groupings and nuclear characteristics. Of all the cell types of invasive squamous cancer of the cervix, these are the most likely to be syncytial, or grouped as clusters with irregular borders (Fig. 11-5). One fourth of the nuclei contain nucleoli, in addition to the usual complement of coarsely granular chromatin (Fig. 11-2, A). In contrast, cells of adenocarcinoma usually occur in smaller groupings, have similar nuclear granularity and almost always contain nucleoli. Despite such differentiating cytologic features, distinction between large-cell, nonkeratinizing squamous cancer and adenocarcinoma of the cervix may be difficult.

Small Cells

These cells may be difficult to identify because of their small size; they have mean nuclear areas only about 1.5 times the size of histiocyte nuclei.[14, 18] Thus, the cytologist must exercise extreme caution in

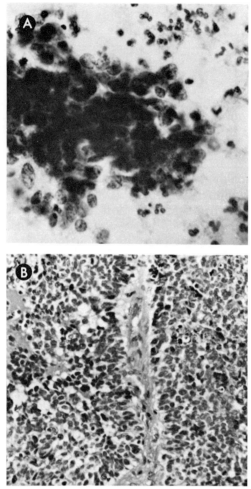

Fig. 11-5. — Nonkeratinizing cells of invasive squamous cell carcinoma. **A,** group of cells from the smear of a patient with large nonkeratinizing squamous cancer. The cells are in a syncytium which has an irregular border. The nuclei are remarkably similar in size and are oval to ellipsoidal in shape. Intrinsic nuclear characteristics of this cell type are shown in better detail in Figure 11-2A. **B,** biopsy of the patient whose smear is shown in **A.** Cells are regular and do not keratinize.

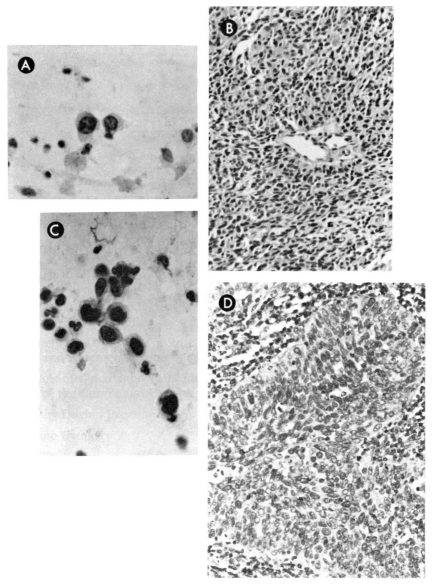

Fig. 11-6. – Small cell invasive cancer. **A**, cervical smear with two small, slightly irregular malignant cells in the center. Nuclei occupy a large percentage of the total cell area and are round with a coarse chromatin pattern. Small nucleoli are seen with difficulty. **B**, histologic section from the same patient as shown in **A**. The small size of the individual cells is readily apparent. **C**, small malignant cells showing greater variation in size and shape of cytoplasm and nucleus than those shown in **A**. Nuclear chromatin, while very coarse, is not "India ink" in character. **D**, histologic section corresponding to the cells depicted in **C**.

screening not to overlook them (Fig. 11-6). When stained optimally* they seldom have the opaque or "India ink" nuclear structure erroneously ascribed to them. Under such conditions, about 20% of small cells also contain nucleoli.

Practical Diagnostic Features for the Cytologic Diagnosis of Invasive Squamous Cervical Cancer

Proper cytologic evaluation of invasive squamous cancer of the cervix depends on analysis of three pertinent features: general cell pattern, malignant cell types and background.

The general cell pattern in smears from invasive cancer reveals a significant hiatus between normal and malignant cells. In these cytosmears, dysplastic cells and cellular types characteristic of in situ cancer are less often observed than they are in cases of in situ cancer. A higher proportion of the cells are often undifferentiated in invasive cancer. On the other hand, predominance of small, keratinizing or undifferentiated cells may, at times, be seen in either invasive or in situ cancer. In such instances, analysis of background smear feature may be important for more precise cytologic diagnosis. Necrosis and degenerated blood are uncommon features of carcinoma in situ; the presence of such background findings is strongly suggestive of an invasive neoplasm. A more accurate diagnosis of a specific cancer type (invasive or in situ) may be made by analysis of all features. Obviously, pertinent clinical data may also be invaluable, in view of the pronounced difference between the two lesions in clinical manifestations.

REFERENCES

1. Boschann, H. W.: Are spindle-shaped squamoid cells suggestive of a distinct type of carcinoma or of a distinct degree of cellular maturity? Acta cytol. 2:272, 1958.
2. deBrux, J., Dupré-Froment, J., and Rauzy, A.: Occurrence of spindle-shaped squamoid cells in dysplasia, Acta cytol. 2:243, 1958.
3. deBrux, J., Dupré-Froment, J., and Rauzy, A.: Occurrence of spindle-shaped squamoid cells in carcinoma in situ, Acta cytol. 2:248, 1958.
4. Gard, P. D., et al.: Comparative cytopathology of in situ cancer of the cervix in the aged, Acta cytol. In press.
5. Graham, R. M., et al.: Definition of spindle-shaped squamoid cells, Acta cytol. 2:208, 1958.
6. Hopman, B. C.: Can carcinoma in situ be differentiated from invasive carcinoma by means of exfoliative cytology? Acta cytol. 5:440, 1961.
7. Jenny, J., and Wacek, A.: Can carcinoma in situ be differentiated from invasive carcinoma by means of exfoliative cytology? Acta cytol. 5:446, 1961.
8. Koss, L. G.: Diagnostic Cytology and Its Histopathologic Bases (2d ed.; Philadelphia and Montreal: J. B. Lippincott Company, 1968).
9. Meisels, A.: An analysis of the vaginal flora as observed on routine VCE smears of 63,870 patients: possible relationship between type of flora and certain cervical atypicalities. Presented at 15th Annual Scientific Meeting of the American Society of Cytology, Denver, Colorado, Oct. 23, 1967.

*Staining is considered optimal when polymorphonuclear leukocytic nuclei show a recognizable chromatin structure.

10. Montalvo-Ruiz, L.: Can carcinoma in situ be differentiated from invasive carcinoma by means of exfoliative cytology? Acta cytol. 5:447, 1961.
11. Okagaki, T., *et al.*: Diagnosis of anaplasia and carcinoma in situ by differential cell counts, Acta cytol. 6:343, 1962.
12. Rappolt, R. T.: The composite high risk cervical cancer candidate, Am. J. Obst. & Gynec. 95:1009, 1966.
13. Reagan, J. W., and Hamonic, M. J.: The cellular pathology in carcinoma in situ, Cancer 9:385, 1956.
14. Reagan, J. W., Hamonic, M. J., and Wentz, W. B.: Analytical study of the cells in cervical squamous-cell cancer, Lab. Invest. 6:241, 1957.
15. Roberts, T. W., and Linkins, T.: Differentiation between intramucosal and invasive carcinoma of the cervix by cytologic smear. It is reliable? Acta cytol. 8:280, 1964.
16. Terzano, G.: Occurrence of spindle-shaped squamoid cells in infections, Acta cytol. 2: 241, 1958.
17. Tweeddale, D. N., *et al.*: Cervical vs. endometrial carcinoma, Obst. & Gynec. 2:623, 1953.
18. Tweeddale, D. N., *et al.*: Giant cells in cervico-vaginal smears, Acta cytol. 12:298, 1968.
19. Wahi, P. N., *et al.*: Intra-epithelial carcinoma of the uterine cervix, Acta Unio internat. contra. cancrum 19:1379, 1963.
20. Wied, G. L.: The potentialities of the smear technique for the differentiation of noninvasive and invasive cervical carcinoma, Am. J. Obst. & Gynec. 71:793, 1956.
21. Wied, G. L., *et al.*: Cytology of invasive cervical carcinoma and carcinoma in situ, Ann. New York Acad. Sc. 97:759, 1962.

CHAPTER 12

The Cytopathology of Microinvasive Squamous Carcinoma of the Cervix

Introduction and Definition

CARCINOMA OF THE CERVIX presumably evolves from epithelium at or near the squamocolumnar junction. Epithelial alterations usually progress from the initial lesion of dysplasia to carcinoma in situ (Fig. 12-1, A) with eventual "flaking off" of small tongues or nests of cells, to yield microinvasive (Fig. 12-1 B, C and D), or early invasive cancer (Fig. 12-1, E), and eventually to clinically overt malignancy. Of the aforementioned, microinvasive, or early invasive, cancer has been the most difficult lesion to define. In the first stage of invasion, individual cells "flake off" (Fig. 12-2), or sharp tongues of cells extend either through the basement membrane of surface or glands – and only rarely into vascular channels.[13, 20] Tongues of cells, connected by a narrow epithelial cord to overlying epithelium, are mostly destined to disintegrate without metastasizing since lymph glands are almost never affected at this stage.[13] This epithelial alteration is common and may be observed in 5% –63% of cases with in situ cancer.[2, 5, 6, 8, 9, 11, 12, 14, 16, 17, 18] Some have designated the change as stage Ia[14] or type Ia_0,[9] but do not include such disease in the spectrum of true "microcarcinoma" (microinvasive or early invasive cancer). Instead, to fulfill that definition, there must be definite early, focal, discrete or confluent stromal invasion, with or without involvement of lymphatic channels. These tumors are entirely microscopic, may measure up to 5 mm. deep and are devoid of clinical or obvious gross pathologic findings. Some have designated them as stage Ia when up to 3 mm. deep,[9] or Ia_2 when up to 5 mm. deep. Rarely are pelvic lymph nodes affected[3, 4] and a uniformly good outcome may be anticipated.[3, 5, 8, 9, 17, 18, 21, 22] Slightly larger, especially symptomatic, cancers do not seem to carry such a favorable prognosis.[7, 9, 10, 15]

We describe here the clinical, pathologic and cytologic findings we

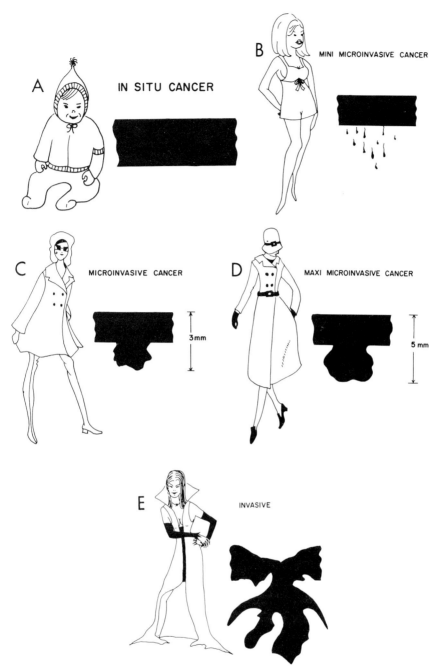

Fig. 12-1. — Artist's conception of the extension of cancer from its earliest in situ to frankly invasive state. The earliest stages of invasion have been subdivided into lesions of progressively greater magnitude: mini microinvasive, microinvasive, and maxi microinvasive. The mini microinvasive cancer (Figs. 12-1B and 12-2) represents the first stage of invasion wherein individual cells "flake off" from carcinoma in situ that involves surface epithelium or gland depths. This lesion seldom penetrates into the stroma for more than 1 or 2 mm. and has biologic behavior like carcinoma in situ. Microinvasive cancers are actually small, discrete invasive squamous carcinomas which extend into the underlying stroma for a distance not exceeding 5 mm. (Figs. 12-1C, and 12-1D and 12-9). The classic invasive cancer extends beyond the aforementioned limits (Fig. 12-1E).

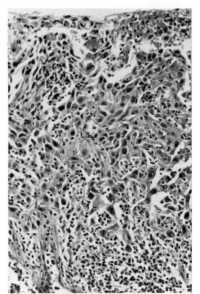

Fig. 12-2. – Photomicrograph showing early penetration of malignant epithelium into underlying stroma, so-called flaking off. This finding is commonly encountered in lesions that are otherwise in situ cancer. H. and E. ×64.

observed to be characteristic of clinically occult squamous cancers of the cervix measuring to 0.5 cm. in depth, based upon a review of 12 cases.

Clinical Features

AGE AND MARITAL STATUS. – Our patients with microinvasive cancer had a mean age of 38.5 years, ranging from age 23 to 51. Two were postmenopausal. Mean age and age range of these patients did not differ significantly from those with in situ cancer in our institution and elsewhere. All patients were or had been married.

PARITY. – All of our patients were multiparous, with an average of 4.83 pregnancies, ranging from 1 – 12. Again, such findings were similar to those from patients with in situ cancer, in our institution and elsewhere.

SYMPTOMS. – Table 12-1 shows that half of the patients had some form of abnormal vaginal bleeding. In no case was it severe, usually consisting of no more than transitory spotting. Bleeding probably reflects the erosion of walls of superficial vasculature (Fig. 12-3). Other

TABLE 12-1.—SYMPTOMS OF MICROINVASIVE CANCER OF THE CERVIX (0.5 CM. OR SMALLER) – 12 PATIENTS

SYMPTOM	NUMBER OF PATIENTS
Bleeding	3
Vaginal discharge & bleeding	3
Vaginal discharge (nonbloody)	3
Pain	3
Asymptomatic	3

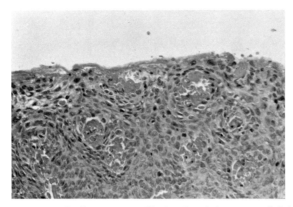

Fig. 12-3.—Photomicrograph showing capillaries involving superficial epithelial layers from an area immediately adjacent to a microinvasive cancer. Rupture of such vascular spaces incident to taking a cervical smear may be responsible for blood seen in smears from patients with microinvasive cancer. H. and E. ×64.

symptoms were of a nonspecific nature such as might accompany the usual forms of chronic cervicitis. A number of patients had a multiplicity of symptoms, accounting for the number of instances recorded in Table 12-1.

APPEARANCE OF THE CERVIX.—In no case was there a clinically demonstrable lesion, substantiating the occult nature of the disease process. Usually, the cervix did not differ significantly on examination from that typical of our general clinic population. In 4 patients the cervix showed an erosion; in 3, it was hypertrophic; in 1, it was clean; and in 4, its appearance was not stated.

Cytologic Characteristics of Associated Non-neoplastic Elements

INFLAMMATION.—All 12 patients had some form of inflammatory response; in most, it was moderate to marked in severity. In general, preserved polymorphonuclear cells predominated, although a few lymphocytes, histiocytes or eosinophils were often present. While inflammatory response was observed more commonly than with in situ carcinoma, it was not sufficiently striking to be a diagnostic feature.

BACTERIAL FLORA.—In over 60% of the slides, an abnormal bacterial flora was present; it consisted primarily of rods or cocci. Of the other 40%, either no bacteria were observed or Döderlein bacilli were apparent. It is apparent that bacterial flora in microinvasive cancer is similar to that encountered in carcinoma in situ.

ERYTHROCYTES.—The smears of slightly over half of the patients contained erythrocytes, usually light to moderate in number, showing various degrees of preservation or degeneration. Red blood cells were not as commonly observed in smears from patients with carcinoma in situ.

TRICHOMONADS. — *Trichomonas vaginalis* was encountered in 2 of the 12 cases of microinvasive cancer (17%).

NECROSIS. — In only 1 case of 12 was there a background that indicated necrosis. Such a finding is similar to the picture of in situ cancer in women of the same age. Apparently, the microinvasive lesion is so small that significant necrosis is uncommon, although small amounts of superficial surface ulceration and inflammatory response are commonly encountered.

MATURATION INDEX. — The maturation index of non-neoplastic cells was that expected for the patients' menstrual status. Similar findings are observed in smears from patients with carcinoma in situ and invasive cancer.

Cellular Patterns Seen in Microinvasive Cancer of the Cervix — Percentage Distribution of Malignant Cell Types

Table 12-2 outlines the cell types observed in microinvasive cervical cancer; cell characteristics have been previously described in detail. In this lesion, as in carcinoma in situ, malignant cells are predominantly isodiametric.[1] However, the most significant differential feature between the two conditions is that the cytologic smears of microinvasive lesions contain nine times the number of large, nonkeratinizing cells (Fig. 12-4) and tend to contain more keratinizing cancer cells (Fig. 12-5) and fewer isodiametric, parabasal-like cells (clustered cancer and parabasal-type cells). Alousi and associates[1] measured atypical cells from microinvasive carcinoma. They found mean nuclear areas to be 89.5 sq. μ; Reagan et al.,[19] recorded mean nuclear areas of large nonkeratinizing cells to be 87.84 sq. μ contrasted to 109.4 sq. μ for cells from in situ cancer.

The predominant malignant cell type shown in Table 12-3 reflects these observations. As expected from findings in Table 12-2, in three quarters of the cases large, nonkeratinizing or keratinizing cancer cells

---

TABLE 12-2. — PERCENTAGE DISTRIBUTION OF CELL TYPES IN AN AGGREGATE OF 12 CASES OF MICROINVASIVE CERVICAL CANCER

CELL TYPE	PER CENT OF TOTAL CELL POPULATION (12 CASES)
Large cell, nonkeratinizing	46*
Keratinizing cancer cell	25
Clustered cancer cell	8*
Small cancer cell	8*
Undifferentiated cancer cell	6
Parabasal cancer cell	4*
Fiber cell	3

*70% of the total cell population is isodiametric.
(This table reflects a composite analysis of the malignant cell types in 12 cases of microinvasive cancer.)

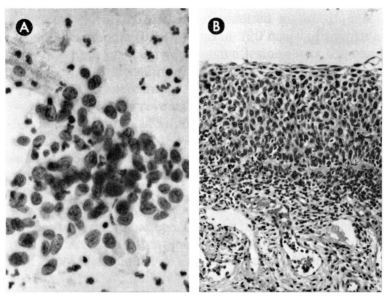

Fig. 12-4.—**A**, large nonkeratinizing malignant cells. These cells were the most commonly encountered malignant cells in cytologic smears from patients with microinvasive cancer. A modest amount of cyanophilic cytoplasm accompanies. The nuclei are round, oval
or ellipsoid and contain finely stippled chromatin separated by vesicular areas. At times,
nuclear chromatin is condensed to form chromocenters or nucleoli. Such cells are commonly arranged in groupings. **B**, histologic counterpart of the cells depicted in **A**. This
area of in situ cancer was immediately adjacent to a zone of microinvasion. In general,
the cells comprising this lesion are of similar size and shape throughout the entire epithelial thickness. H. and E. ×64.

predominated. The most remarkable observation is that only one case
had a predominance of clustered cancer or parabasal-type cells, in
sharp contrast with smears from in situ cancers, whether in younger or
older women, where that finding was common.

Of the 6 cases characterized by large, nonkeratinizing cell types, 5
showed 80% – 100% of these types in the cell population and they were
accompanied by cells that were parabasal type, fiber or undifferentiated, not exceeding 10% for each of these types. In the sixth case,
large, nonkeratinizing cells comprised 60%, associated with 40% of
clustered cancer cells.

In the cases showing mostly keratinizing cancer cells, two showed
90% of that cell type with 10% fiber cells in each. The third case had

TABLE 12-3.—PREDOMINANT MALIGNANT CELL TYPES PER CASE
FROM MICROINVASIVE CERVICAL CANCER

CELL TYPE	NUMBER OF CASES
Large cell, nonkeratinizing	6
Keratinizing cancer cell	3
Small cancer cell	1
Clustered cancer cell	1
Undifferentiated cancer cell	1

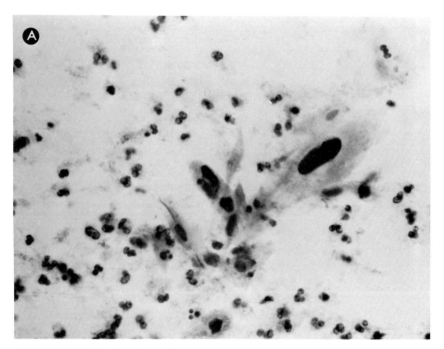

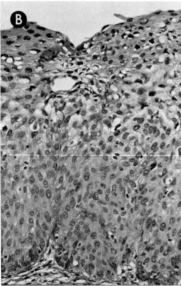

Fig. 12-5. – **A**, keratinizing cancer cells, the second most common cell type observed in smears representative of microinvasive cancer. These cells are characteristically irregular and have a variable amount of eosinophilic cytoplasm. Nuclei are also irregular and contain a complement of very heavily clumped chromatin. Nucleoli are rarely seen. **B**, histologic section of an area of in situ cancer, adjacent to a microinvasive focus, showing a keratinizing pattern to correspond with the cytologic pattern depicted in **A**. There is loss of cell polarity throughout the entire epithelial thickness. Nuclei in cells near the surface are more irregular and stain more intensely than those in deeper layers. H. and E. ×64.

60% keratinizing cancer cells with the remainder clustered cancer and parabasal-type cells in equal numbers.

The smear with small cancer cells showed that cell type exclusively (Fig. 12-6).

The single instance of predominating clustered cancer cells manifested 40% of that cell type and 30% each of large, nonkeratinizing and keratinizing cancer cells (Fig. 12-7).

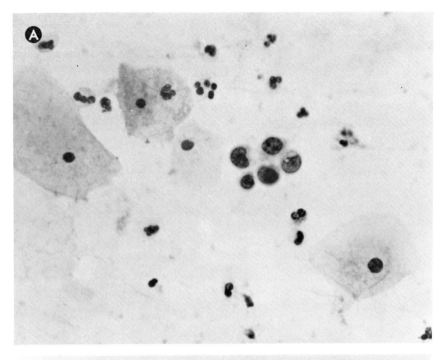

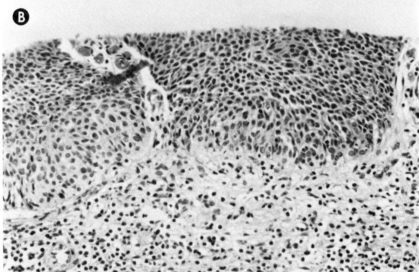

Fig. 12-6. — **A**, small malignant cells, an uncommon cell type in smears from cases of microinvasive cancer. These small, round, or oval cells have scant cytoplasm. Nuclei, which correspond to over-all cell shape, are composed of coarsely clumped chromatin. Nucleoli are not uncommon. **B**, histologic section of an area of in situ cancer composed of small malignant cells immediately adjacent to a microinvasive focus. The corresponding cytology is in **A**. The constituent cells are quite small and are fairly regular in size throughout the entire epithelial thickness. H. and E. ×64.

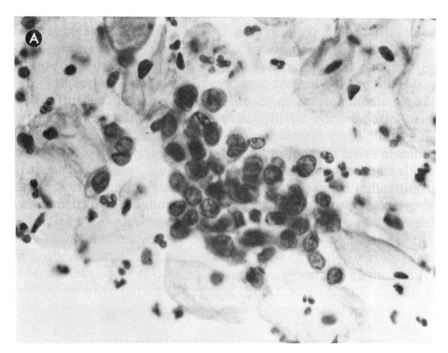

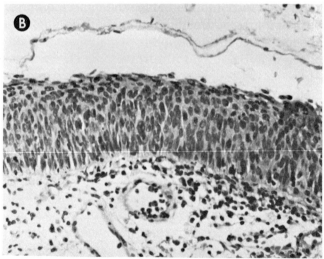

Fig. 12-7.—**A**, malignant parabasal cells in smears from a patient with microinvasive cancer. This is an uncommonly observed pattern in smears representing microinvasive cancer. In many respects, these cells are similar to large, nonkeratinizing cells. However, malignant parabasal cells usually have less cytoplasm, more coarsely clumped nuclear chromatin and fewer chromocenters, or nucleoli, than those that are large nonkeratinizing. **B**, histologic section of zone of in situ cancer composed of parabasal cells, adjacent to a microinvasive focus. In general, the histologic pattern is similar to that of the large, nonkeratinizing type of epithelioma. However, the more compact appearance of the nuclei in this figure, in contrast with Figure 12-4A, probably represents a decrease in nuclear/cytoplasmic ratio. H. and E. ×64.

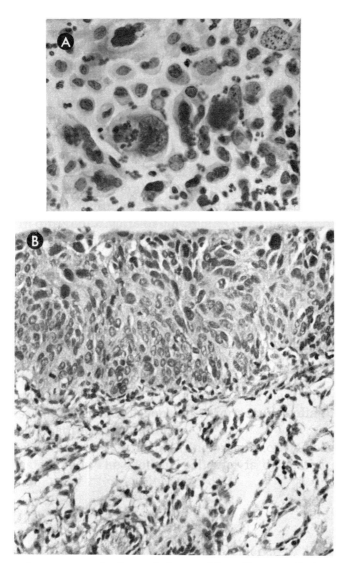

Fig. 12-8. — **A,** the uncommonly observed pleomorphic malignant cells from smears of an individual with microinvasive cancer. Variation in cell size and shape is obvious. Similarly, nuclear shape, size and chromatin pattern differ markedly from one cell to another. In most instances, one might erroneously diagnose such a smear to represent frankly invasive cancer, unless alerted by a clean background which shows no necrotic debris. **B,** histologic section of in situ cancer adjacent to a microinvasive focus from the same case shown in **A.** The variability in the cells composing the histologic picture is easily appreciated. This pattern is ominous in appearance; however, it is unknown whether its biologic potential differs from other types of microinvasive cancer. H. and E. ×64.

In the 1 case with a maximum number of undifferentiated cells (Fig. 12-8), they constituted 60% of the cell population, associated with 30% of keratinizing cancer and 10% fiber cells.

General Spectrum of Neoplastic and Non-neoplastic Cellular Constituents from Smears of Microinvasive Cancer

General cellular constituents per slide in cases of microinvasive cancer closely parallel findings noted with in situ neoplasia. For example, normal cells averaged 60%, dysplastic 16.6% and malignant 23.4%, while comparable findings were 50%, 15% and 35%, respectively, in slides from patients with in situ cancer. The only apparent feature of differential value is that microinvasive lesions contain a greater number of malignant cells that are of a less differentiated type. However, in any single case such an observation is probably valueless.

Correlated Cytohistologic Patterns Observed in Microinvasive Cancer of the Cervix

This lesion has been previously defined as a discrete, invasive squamous cancer measuring less than 0.5 cm. in depth of penetration beyond the basement membrane. Careful analysis reveals close accord between histologic and cytologic qualities. For example, cytologic prep-

Fig. 12-9.—A microinvasive focus adjacent to the surface lesion depicted in Figure 12-7B. Notice how the cell type has changed; individual cells not only have acquired more cytoplasm, but cell groups have formed into whorls, representing squamous pearls. This finding was observed in at least one half of microinvasive cancers, regardless of the surface cell type. H. and E. ×64.

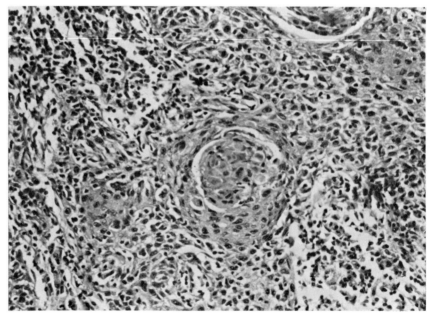

arations will show that most microinvasive cancers are composed of regular, round, oval or ellipsoid cells. An equivalent histologic picture is classically associated with carcinoma in situ that almost always accompanies as a major component of the picture. The associated carcinoma in situ almost always affects glands. The histologic pattern of the microinvasive lesion parallels its cytologic counterpart and is composed of regular cells that are either large nonkeratinizing or, rarely, of clustered cancer type. At other times, the lesion as observed in sections may consist of cells that are small and irregular, or larger, with or without evidence of cytoplasmic keratinization. These varying pictures reflect cytologic patterns that are of small cell, undifferentiated or keratinizing, respectively. Regardless of the cell type of the in situ lesion, at least one half of these lesions show keratinizing tendencies as they invade (Fig. 12-9), also observed by Christopherson & Parker.[3] Two of our patients had slight leukoplakia of the carcinoma in situ associated with the microinvasive lesion.

Vascular Involvement

Table 12-4 shows that 5 of the 12 cases (42%) had discrete intravascular segments of tumor (Fig. 12-10). The vascular spaces are presumably lymphatic, since they never appeared to contain erythrocytes. The

Fig. 12-10.—A small focus of vascular involvement in the area of invasion adjacent to the surface lesion depicted in Figure 12-6B. A small group of malignant cells are within a small vascular space, presumably a lymphatic. This is not tantamount to more distant embolism as none of the 5 cases with such involvement had nodal metastases or have had recurrent tumor, either locally or in more distant sites. H. and E. ×160.

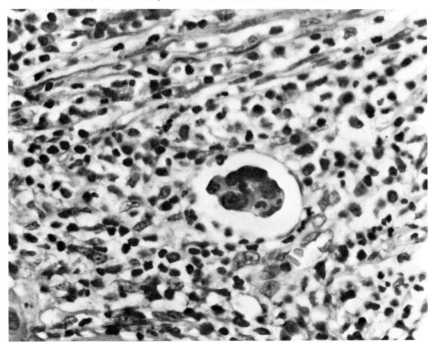

TABLE 12-4.—VASCULAR INVOLVEMENT IN MICROINVASIVE
CERVICAL CANCER (12 CASES)*

DEPTH OF LESION (MM.)	NO. OF CASES	VASCULAR INVOLVEMENT
1	2	$\dfrac{+}{1}$
2	7	3
4	3	1

*Our experience now encompasses 17 cases of which 6 (35%) showed vascular involvement. Of 10 cases with pelvic lymph node dissections, none have shown metastatic neoplasm.

presence of intravascular tumor is not synonymous with embolization in our experience, although such a finding has been uncommonly noted.[3, 4] On follow-up of 6 to 30 months after diagnosis, no patient has shown signs or symptoms of recurrent or residual malignancy.

Practical Diagnostic Features for the Cytologic Diagnosis of Microinvasive Carcinoma of the Cervix

Little difficulty is experienced in categorizing as malignant without qualification smears which are obtained from patients subsequently shown to have microinvasive cancer. However, we experience great difficulty in specifying accurately the correct tissue phase from smear study alone. In most instances, the cellular findings do not differ from those associated with in situ cancer. However, about one fourth of smears contain isodiametric cells combined with those that are undifferentiated, suggesting the possibility of microinvasion. If undifferentiated malignant cells are combined with blood, a cytodiagnosis of invasive malignancy is likely.

REFERENCES

1. Alousi, M. A., et al.: Microinvasive carcinoma and inflammatory lesions of the cervix uteri: histologic and cytologic differentiation, Acta cytol. 11:132, 1967.
2. Boyes, D. A., Fidler, H. K., and Lock, D. R.: Significance of in situ carcinoma of the uterine cervix, Brit. M. J. 203:5273, 1962.
3. Christopherson, W. M., and Parker, J. E.: Microinvasive carcinoma of the uterine cervix: a clinical-pathological study, Cancer 17:1123, 1964.
4. Decker, W. H.: Minimal invasive carcinoma of the cervix with lymph node metastasis. Report of a case, Am. J. Obst. & Gynec.72:1116, 1956.
5. Fennell, R. H., Jr.: Carcinoma in situ of cervix with early invasive changes, Cancer 8: 302, 1955.
6. Fennell, R. H., Jr.: Carcinoma in situ of the uterine cervix: a report of 118 cases, Cancer 9:374, 1956.
7. Fidler, H. K., and Boyd, J. R.: Occult invasive squamous carcinoma of the cervix, Cancer 13:764, 1960.
8. Fidler, H. K., and Boyes, D. A.: Patterns of early invasion from intraepithelial carcinoma of the cervix, Cancer 12:673, 1959.
9. Frick, H. C., et al.: Early invasive cancer of the cervix, Am. J. Obst. & Gynec. 85:926, 1963.
10. Friedell, G. H., and Graham, J. B.: Regional lymph node involvement in small carcinoma of the cervix, Surg. Gynec. & Obst. 108:513, 1959.

11. Gusberg, S. B.: Newer concepts of early stages of carcinoma of cervix and their clinical recognition, M. Clin. North America 35:847, 1951.

12. Gusberg, S. B., Fish, S. A., and Wang, Y. Y.: Growth patterns of cervical cancer, Obst. & Gynec. 2:557, 1953.

13. Hamperl, H.: Definition and classification of the so-called carcinoma in situ, Obst. & Gynec. 2:2, 1953.

14. Kottmeier, H. L.: Carcinoma of the cervix, a study of its initial stages, Acta obst. et gynec. scandinav. 38:522, 1959.

15. Kottmeier, H. L., *et al.*: Histopathological Problems Concerning the Early Diagnosis of Carcinoma of the Cervix. Experiences From 2,432 Cases of Carcinoma of the Cervix From the Radiumhemmet, 1949–1954, in Wolstenholme, G. E. W., and O'Conner, M. (eds): *Cancer of the Cervix. Diagnosis of Early Forms*, Ciba Foundation Study Group 3 (Boston: Little, Brown & Company, 1959), pp. 20–27.

16. Latour, J. P. A.: Results in the management of preclinical cancer of the cervix, Tr. Am. A. Obst. & Gynec. 71:99, 1960.

17. Latour, J. P. A., Brown, L. B., and Turnbull, L. A.: Preclinical carcinoma of the cervix, Am. J. Obst. & Gynec. 74:354, 1957.

18. Morton, D. G.: Incipient cervical carcinoma, Am. J. Obst. & Gynec. 90:64, 1964.

19. Reagan, J. W., Hamonic, M. J., and Wentz, W. B.: Analytical study of the cells in cervical squamous-cell cancer, Lab. Invest. 6:241, 1957.

20. Stoddard, L. D.: Problem of Carcinoma in Situ with Reference to Human Cervix Uteri, in McManus, J. F. A. (ed.): *Progress in Fundamental Medicine* (Philadelphia: Lea & Febiger, 1952), pp. 203–260.

21. Stoddard, L. D., Erickson, C. C., and Howard, H. L.: Further studies on the histogenesis of intra-epithelial carcinoma and early invasive carcinoma of the cervix uteri, Am. J. Path. 26:679, 1950.

22. Way, S.: Microinvasive carcinoma of the cervix, Acta cytol. 8:14, 1964.

CHAPTER 13

Cytopathology of Cervical Adenocarcinoma

CERVICAL ADENOCARCINOMA is a neoplasm that usually originates from gland cells of the endocervix, although a lesser number arise from mesonephric remnants in the lateral aspects of this organ.[2] The neoplasm is one-twentieth as common but is more malignant than squamous cancer of the cervix, the latter most likely because of its more occult character during earlier stages of genesis.[8] Evidence also indicates that, stage* for stage, adenocarcinoma of the cervix is a more serious lesion than squamous cancer, in part a reflection of decreased radiosensitivity of the former.[8]

General Clinical and Pathologic Characteristics

The typical patient with cervical adenocarcinoma is slightly postmenopausal in age, as with invasive squamous cell carcinoma. Unlike squamous cell carcinoma, there is no racial predilection and no significance can be ascribed to early coitus or parity. Presenting signs and symptoms are similar to those for squamous cancer: atypical vaginal discharge or bleeding, pain, frequency or dysuria or, with advanced lesions, manifestations of extrapelvic spread. The cancer is most commonly papillary, but ulcerative lesions are almost as frequent. As with squamous cancer, adenocarcinoma may be at any clinical stage when initially detected. Histologically, all grades of malignancy may be observed, but grade II (on the basis of I–IV†) lesions are more frequent. Microscopic patterns are variable, some being ductlike, others papillary,

---

*Stage refers to the extent of disease as determined by clinical examination. There are four clinical stages. For example, stage I lesions are confined to the cervix, while those that are stage IV have spread beyond the confines of the pelvis and/or have invaded the bladder or rectum. Prognosis decreases with an increase in clinical stage.

†Grading is determined by studying histologic sections. Tumors of well-differentiated nature mimic cells of origin and are graded I or II. Those poorly differentiated tumors bear little or no resemblance to cells of origin and are graded III or IV. As a general rule, grade and stage do not correspond.

with constituent cells being either small, large or mucous (colloid) in character.[8]

In Situ and Microinvasive Endocervical Adenocarcinoma – General Concepts

Since it is more frequent and more easily detectable at an early stage, squamous cancer has received the lion's share of attention regarding genesis and early diagnosis by cytohistologic studies. However, years ago, transitional stages from normal to neoplastic columnar cells were described[3, 15, 20] and, more recently, very early, at times in situ, cervical adenocarcinomas have been documented.[1, 14] For example, Abell and Gosling[1] described 10 cases of noninfiltrative gland cell carcinomas of the cervix, 7 of which were restricted to a polyp (Fig. 13-1). Of particular interest is the recording of endocervical in situ adenocarcinoma in combination with a second epithelial neoplasm in the female genital tract.[1, 5, 6, 12] In 2 instances, an associated adenocarcinoma in situ of the endometrium was recorded and, in another 2, squamous cell epithelioma in situ of the cervix was present.[1, 12]

There have also been examples of early invasive cervical adenocarcinoma with transitional areas with a second genital malignancy. Friedell and McKay[6] described 0.5 cm. in diameter invasive adenocarcinoma on the anterior cervical lip associated with an anaplastic carcinoma of the posterior lip. An instance of early adenosquamous carcinoma of the cervix with transitional zones has been recorded,[5] as well as a number of cases of cervical adenosquamous carcinoma in situ.[16] Table 13-1 records our experience with 4 minimally invasive gland-cell cancers of the cervix; it is of interest that 2 patients also had lesions representing either dysplasia or in situ squamous cancer (Fig. 13-2). The aforementioned presents the cytologist with a confusing pattern of atypical glandular and squamous cells. Difficulties in the early diagnosis of cervical adenocarcinoma are further compounded by the difficult cytology of the first blush of malignancy, as well as potential lack of recognition due to its isolated intraglandular location.

All of our early, subclinical cervical adenocarcinomas were of grade I malignancy. However, not all grade I lesions are of early clinical stage or extent of spread. In fact, there is little relationship between histologic grade and clinical stage of cervical cancer, whether adenocarcinoma or squamous. In the text to follow, neoplastic cellular morphology of cervical adenocarcinoma is described to correspond primarily to histologic grade. Non-neoplastic smear findings are primarily described in relationship to clinical stage. The cellular pattern of cancers of lesser grades of malignancy more closely mimic parent cells than those representing high-grade tumors.

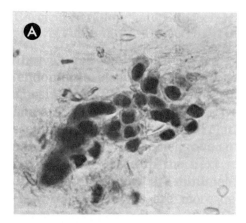

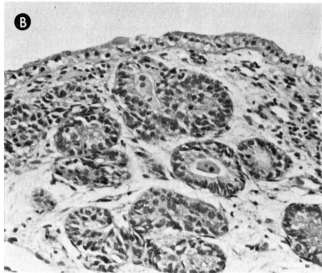

Fig. 13-1. – Adenocarcinoma, grade I, which was confined to an endocervical polyp. **A**, closely grouped small cells in a cervical smear. They have hyperchromatic nuclei with an altered nuclear/cytoplasmic ratio. Some cells (not shown in this photomicrograph) had prominent, large cytoplasmic vacuoles. **B**, histologic section from the patient whose cells are shown in **A**. Variance from normal cervical glands is shown by smaller gland size, altered nuclear/cytoplasmic ratio and nuclear hyperchromasia.

TABLE 13-1. – SUBCLINICAL CERVICAL ADENOCARCINOMAS

CASE	AGE	RACE	CLIN. LESION	RX	F-UP	G.	P.
1	36	W	None	Hyst.	4 mos.	?	2
2(D)	33	W	1 cm.	Hyst.	3½ yrs.	3	2
3	37	W	None	Rad.	2½ yrs.	7	7
4(D)	34	W	Eroded	Hyst.	None	6	5
	35					5+	4

(D) Associated dysplasia.

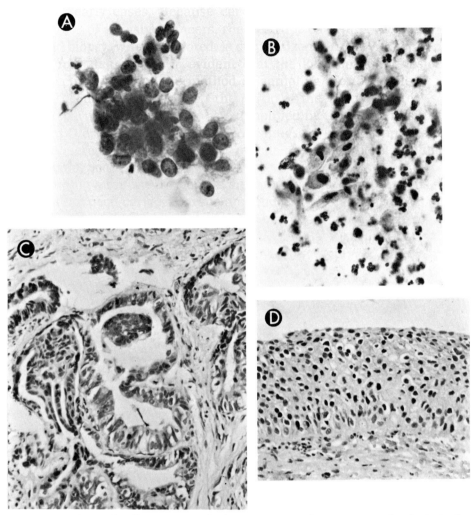

Fig. 13-2.—Cervical collison tumor of adenocarcinoma plus squamous dysplasia in the same patient. **A**, cells from a smear from the adenocarcinoma portion. **B**, cells from a smear from the dysplastic component. **C**, histologic section of the low-grade adenocarcinoma. **D**, histologic section of the separate dysplastic process.

Non-neoplastic Cellular Characteristics of Cervical Adenocarcinoma

This section describes the relationship of stage to certain non-neoplastic findings in smears from cervical adenocarcinoma. Erythrocytes, inflammatory cells and necrosis are detailed for the most part with respect to clinical stage, as they are at times related.

ERYTHROCYTES. — A small number of erythrocytes may be observed in all stages and grades of endocervical adenocarcinoma. In general, patients with more advanced disease have a greater number of erythrocytes. These cells may be preserved or degenerated, depending on how recently bleeding occurred prior to taking the smear. Erythrocytes are

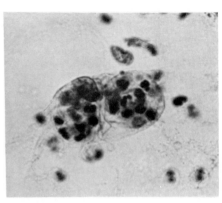

Fig. 13-3. — Cervical adenocarcinoma, grade II. Cells from a cervical smear show cannibalism of polymorphonuclear leukocytes. This finding is less common in cervical adenocarcinoma than in endometrial adenocarcinoma. It is conjectural as to whether the cancer cells are eating the leukocytes or vice versa.

so commonly present in smears from neoplastic and non-neoplastic uterine processes that they are more of nuisance value than of diagnostic significance, often obscuring the presence of or diluting malignant cells.

INFLAMMATORY CELLS. — There is no relationship between the number of inflammatory cells and the stage of cervical adenocarcinoma. For example, it is possible to have a marked inflammatory response in stage I lesions and none in a stage III cancer; the opposite, however, may also be true. The inflammatory response usually consists of polymorphonuclear leukocytes. Presence of numerous leukocytes and of necrotic debris do not parallel one another; it is possible that a marked polymorphonuclear response may be unattended by the presence of necrotic debris. Intracellular polymorphonuclear leukocytes are seldom encountered, their presence more commonly indicating a tumor originating in the endometrium (Fig. 13-3).[13]

NECROSIS. — Necrosis is an unusual finding in smears from stage 0 and I cervical adenocarcinomas. In lesions of progressively higher stage, necrosis is encountered more commonly; in at least one quarter of advanced cases, a necrotic background can be anticipated. Because mucus is present, the background in cervical adenocarcinoma is not as commonly "dirty" as it is in smears from overt squamous carcinoma.[12]

Similarly, diathesis* is less common in endocervical adenocarcinoma than in endometrial adenocarcinoma. On the other hand, diathesis is more frequent with dedifferentiated cervical adenocarcinoma.[14]

Neoplastic Cellular Characteristics of Cervical Adenocarcinoma

GENERAL FEATURES. — Cellular characteristics of endocervical adenocarcinoma vary widely. In some instances, they closely mimic normal endocervical cells in size and configuration, differing only subtly, e.g., as slightly enlarged nuclei with minimal hyperchromasia (Fig. 13-4).[11]

Refer to Chapter 15, "The Cytopathology of Endometrial Adenocarcinoma" for definition.

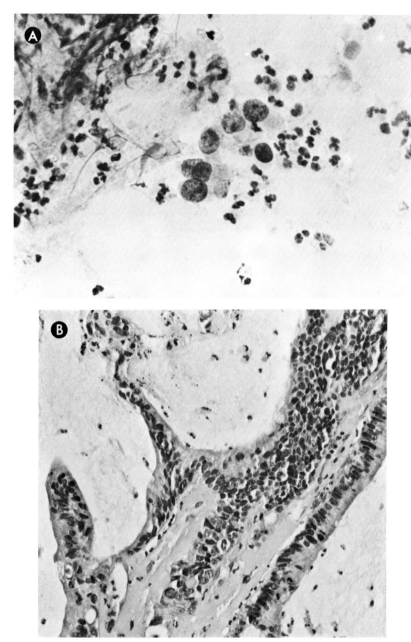

Fig. 13-4. – Cervical adenocarcinoma, grade I. **A,** cells from a cervical smear which are larger than normal endocervical cells. The nuclei occupy a slightly larger percentage of the cell area and nuclear hyperchromasia is subtle. Nucleoli are not unduly prominent. These cells present a very difficult diagnostic problem. **B,** histologic section of the cervical biopsy from the patient whose cells are shown in **A.** The tumor produced considerable mucus, although the cells do not display prominent vacuoles.

At the other end of the spectrum, extremely pleomorphic cytologic patterns cause difficulty in differentiation from large, nonkeratinizing squamous cancer, and even certain sarcomas, even though cells are ovoid in configuration. For the most part, however, cervical adenocarcinomas are cytologically recognizable; since most are of higher grades of malignancy than endometrial adenocarcinoma, they can generally be differentiated from the usually well-differentiated cells of those cancers (Fig. 13-5).

CELL NUMBER AND GROUPINGS. — Smears from endocervical adenocar-

Fig. 13-5. — Cervical adenocarcinoma, grade III. **A,** cell from a smear which displays three features of cells from high-grade lesions. The cell is large, the nucleus occupies over half of the total cell area and the nucleolus is prominent. See Figure 13-8 which is from the same case. **B,** histologic section of the tumor of the patient whose cell is shown in **A.**

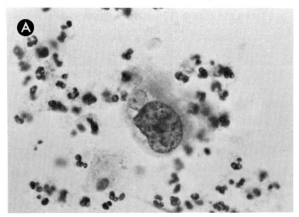

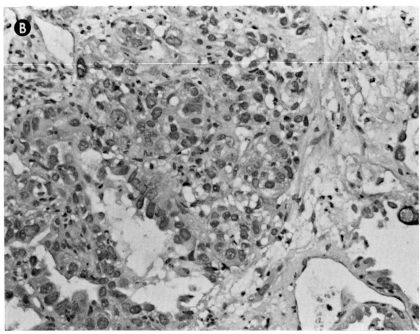

cinoma usually contain fewer malignant cells than are seen in smears from patients with squamous cancer of that organ.[10] Cells in smears from cervical adenocarcinoma are present in greater numbers than in smears from patients with endometrial adenocarcinoma. The latter reflects the rule that by increasing the distance of collection from a tumor site, fewer malignant cells are seen and diagnostic accuracy decreases. The number of cells in smears from cervical adenocarcinoma is not related to the histologic grade of the neoplasm.[14] This is undoubtedly because grade and stage are not related in this cancer.

Cells scraped from endocervical adenocarcinoma are more commonly observed in groupings, though not to the degree seen with endometrial adenocarcinoma. Up to one half of malignant cells may appear singly. In general, tumors of higher grade contain more single neoplastic cells, but notable exceptions are encountered, making this observation of limited diagnostic value in each instance.

Cellular Characteristics of Low-Grade Cervical Adenocarcinoma

Smears from these cancers have cells that vary in size from those slightly smaller to slightly larger than normal endocervical cells. Marked variation in cellular configuration is unusual, with most cancer cells resembling each other in size and general outline. The cells are ordinarily cuboidal to columnar in configuration, mimicking the parent tissue. As previously indicated, cells are more likely to be observed in groupings, and acinar arrangements are not uncommon (Fig. 13-6). Groupings contain from three to hundreds of nuclei arranged in a non-syncytial manner. These groupings are characteristically sharply outlined, quite unlike the irregular outlines seen in groupings common to squamous cancer. The cytoplasm stains either lightly cyanophilic or in indeterminate hues, using EA 36 as the cytoplasmic stain. Others[14] utilizing EA 65 cytoplasmic stain have observed predominately eosinophilic cytoplasm. It is noteworthy that with EA 36 the cytoplasm of benign, hyperplastic endocervical cells is commonly eosinophilic. Cytoplasmic vacuoles are common in low-grade cervical adenocarcinomas. They may be present as a single large vacuole mimicking those in normal endocervical cells, or they may be more numerous and smaller (Fig. 13-7).

All cells demonstrate a reversal of the normal nuclear/cytoplasmic ratio, i.e., the rounded nucleus occupies a proportionally larger percentage of total cell area than normal cells of the endocervix (Figs. 13-4, A, 13-7, A and 13-7, B). This finding in low-grade cervical adenocarcinomas may be subtle, necessitating careful analysis. Nuclear chromatin is coarser than that of normal endocervical cells but is not unusually dense, so that nuclei are often distinctly vesicular. Nuclei may be dis-

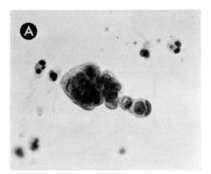

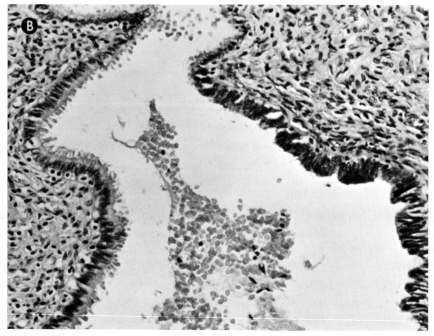

Fig. 13-6.—Cervical adenocarcinoma, grade I. **A,** tightly grouped cluster of cells from a cervicovaginal smear. Malignant changes are subtle and the nuclear/cytoplasmic ratio is minimally altered. Tumors of low-grade malignancies have smaller cells, such as those shown here, than those representing less well-differentiated cancers. **B.** histologic section from the patient in **A.** Note that the right side of the gland is lined by malignant cells, whereas the lining cells on the left side appear normal. Such transitional areas are quite common in early cervical carcinomas.

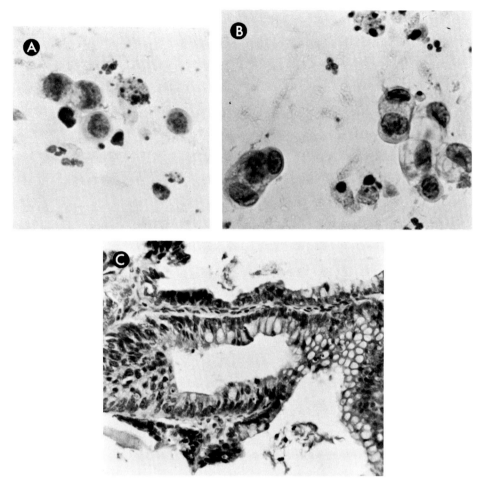

Fig. 13-7. – Cervical adenocarcinoma, grade I. **A** and **B**, these cells from a smear show two significant features: nuclear karyorrhexis, a degenerative phenomenon, is present; and a vesicular nuclear chromatin pattern with moderately prominent nucleoli is evident. The latter is a prominent feature of low-grade cervical adenocarcinoma. **C**, histologic section of the cervical biopsy from the patient whose cells are shown in **A** and **B**. The prominent, large intracytoplasmic vacuoles evident in the tissue section were seen with difficulty in the smears.

torted and assume a crescent shape due to adjacent cells or cytoplasmic vacuoles. Nucleoli, a common feature of adenocarcinoma, are ordinarily small, regular and centrally located. In these carcinomas, they may be difficult to see and careful focusing is a must.

Cellular Characteristics of High-Grade (Undifferentiated) Cervical Adenocarcinoma

The aforementioned cell changes are all accentuated in smears from high-grade cervical adenocarcinomas. For example, these cells are generally larger than those of low-grade adenocarcinoma; indeed, the higher the grade, the larger the cell (Fig. 13-5, A). The cells vary in individual size. Irregular, large, syncytial groupings are more common than in low-grade cancers, in part a reflection of more indistinct cell borders (Figs. 13-5, B and 13-8). Contrasting with low-grade neoplasia, when groupings occur they commonly contain a larger number of nuclei, with up to 500 nuclei per group. Smears from high-grade lesions also tend to contain a greater number of singly occurring cells than those from low-grade adenocarcinomas. The cytoplasm stains a cyanophilic, gray or greenish color, seldom contains prominent vacuoles but is usually granular or finely vacuolated.[14]

A pronounced reversal of the normal nuclear/cytoplasmic ratio causes the nucleus to occupy a still larger percentage of total cell area than that of low-grade adenocarcinomas. Reagan and Ng[14] have calculated the nuclear area of about 50% of total cell area. Nuclear chromatin is significantly hyperchromatic because of uneven clumping of chromatin, contrasting with the fine chromatin clumping of low-grade cancers (Fig. 13-9). Due to dense chromatin clumping in less well-differentiated cancers, the vesicular character of the nucleus is often lost. Nuclei may also be distorted and assume a crescent shape. There are seldom more than two nucleoli, often more prominent and irregular than those

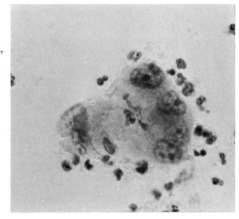

Fig. 13-8.—Cervical adenocarcinoma, grade III. Cells, from a cervical smear, are arranged in a syncytium. They are large, have disproportionately enlarged nuclei, and the cytoplasm is finely granular. Nucleoli are prominent. These findings are not commonly encountered in smears of cells from low-grade cervical adenocarcinoma. Figure 13-5 is from the same case.

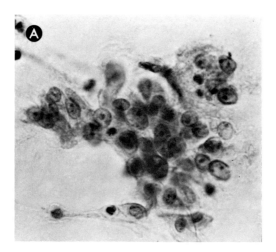

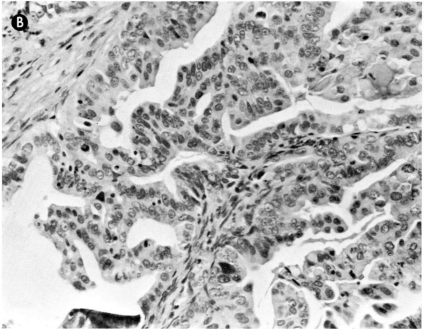

Fig. 13-9.—Cervical adenocarcinoma, grade II. **A,** cells from a smear from the same patient as Figure 13-3. Nucleoli are more prominent than in many grade I adenocarcinomas and the nuclear/cytoplasmic ratio shows greater deviation toward the abnormal. **B,** histologic section of the lesion.

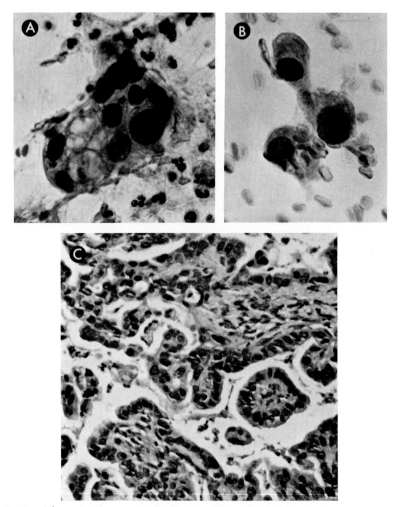

Fig. 13-10.—Adenocarcinoma, grade II. **A** and **B**, cells from a smear are arranged in a syncytial manner, show nuclear size variation, significant hyperchromasia and marked nuclear/cytoplasmic ratio alteration—all features that are not ordinarily found in grade I adenocarcinoma. **C**, histologic section of the cervix of the patient whose cells are shown in **A** and **B**. Cellular pleomorphism is evident, particularly when compared to the grade I adenocarcinoma cells in Figures 13-1, 13-4, 13-6 and 13-7.

observed in low-grade adenocarcinomas (Fig. 13-10). The presence of micronucleoli and macronucleoli in the same nucleus is a highly diagnostic malignant feature. However, this finding is not confined to cervical adenocarcinomas and may be observed in high-grade adenocarcinomas from other sites, or, less commonly, with certain large, nonkeratinizing squamous cancers and some sarcomas.

Cellular Patterns of Adenoacanthoma

An adenoacanthoma is a cervical adenocarcinoma, usually with malignant and, less commonly, benign squamous components. This find-

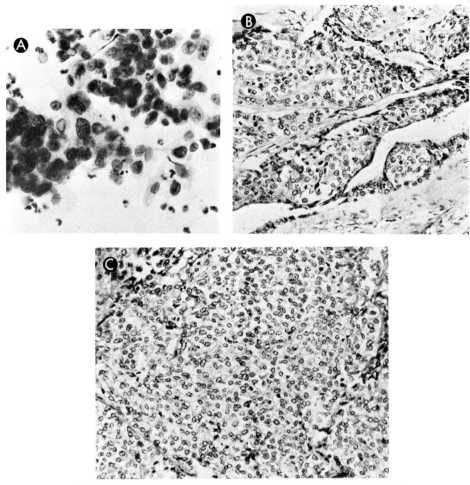

Fig. 13-11. – "Mixed" carcinoma of the cervix, i.e., combined cancers of the squamous and glandular epithelium. **A**, cells from a cervical smear. The squamous component on the right blends into glandular-appearing cells to the left presenting a most difficult diagnostic problem. In our experience, correct cytodiagnosis is often made by hindsight. **B**, histologic section, from the cervix of the same patient as in **A**, which shows irregular gland formation. **C**, another histologic section of the same patient which shows that the tumor is a cross between adenocarcinoma and large nonkeratinizing squamous cancer.

ing may be seen in a large number of cervical adenocarcinomas,[4] especially those associated with pregnancy.[7] Previous observations indicate that only by careful study of adenocarcinomas is it possible to identify such high percentages with squamous elements.[18] If the squamous component is malignant, the lesion is designated adenoacanthoma with malignant squamous component. Others[14] have called this a "mixed carcinoma" or "double epidermoid and columnar carcinoma."[19] This variety of tumor is particularly difficult to diagnose correctly by purely cytologic means. We agree with von Haam[19] that the malignant glandular component may be misinterpreted as an undifferentiated squamous cell. The squamous component is ordinarily of the large, nonkeratinizing variety, which may, at times, simulate cells of high-grade cervical adenocarcinoma. Only if a distinctly malignant glandular pattern is associated with a second component recognizable as a variant of squamous cancer should one suggest a diagnosis of adenoacanthoma with malignant squamous component (mixed carcinoma) by cytologic means alone (Fig. 13-11).

Adenoacanthoma of the cervix with a benign squamous component is an unusual neoplasm. Our experience dictates that it is not ordinarily possible to make this diagnosis cytologically. The association of squamous carcinoma in situ or dysplasia with minimally invasive adenocarcinoma has been noted above. These are not closely combined, but are collison tumors; characteristics of both cell types may be recognized by cytologic means.

Cellular Patterns of Mesonephric Adenocarcinoma (Gartner Duct Origin)

This is a rare variant of cervical adenocarcinoma, recognized in less than 1% of all cervical malignancies.[2] The cells are morphologically variable and may resemble those of tubal adenocarcinoma to undifferentiated cells with dark round nuclei and a small rim of cytoplasm.[2]

Endocervical Adenocarcinoma: Differential Diagnosis

Table 13-2 lists significant features that differentiate various types of lesions. It is pertinent that no single cell characteristic is diagnostic. Experience gained by careful cytohistologic correlation is necessary to differentiate some of the subtle nuances of these lesions.

TABLE 13-2.—SALIENT DIFFERENTIAL CYTOLOGIC FEATURES BETWEEN ENDOCERVICAL ADENOCARCINOMA, ENDOMETRIAL ADENOCARCINOMA, INFLAMMATORY ENDOCERVICAL HYPERTROPHY AND SQUAMOUS CARCINOMA[9, 13, 14]

CELL CHARACTERISTIC	TYPE OF LESION			
	Endocervical Ca.	Endometrial Ca.	Endocervical Hyper.	Squamous Ca.
Number of cells	Many	Few	Moderate	Many
Cell groupings	Grouped or singly	Characteristically grouped	Groupings in focal areas	Grouped or singly occurring
Cell size	Large	Moderate to small	Large	Small
Cytoplasm	More granular, vacuoles less commonly discrete or fine	More discrete vacuoles or finely vacuolated	Large vacuoles or granular	No vacuoles, granular
Nuclear/ cytoplasmic ratio	Markedly altered (increase)	Less markedly altered (increase)	Normal or decreased	Markedly altered (increased)
Nucleus	Coarsely granular chromatin	Less coarsely granular chromatin	Normal chromatin	Clumped chromatin
Background	Mucoid	Diathesis common	Usually numerous PMN's; diathesis rare	Dirty; diathesis unusual

Endocervical adenocarcinoma can ordinarily be differentiated from endometrial adenocarcinoma by the following:

1. Both show characteristics of glandular neoplasia, but cells from endocervical adenocarcinoma are generally more pleomorphic. This is reflected by the greater cell size and disproportionately large nuclear size of endocervical cancers.

2. Endocervical adenocarcinoma has more malignant-appearing and larger nuclei, commonly containing multiple nucleoli.

3. Endometrial cancers often contain cytoplasmic vacuoles, but those of the endocervix less commonly show this feature.

4. Endometrial adenocarcinoma is characterized by cellular spreads with fewer cells, but, when present, cells are more distinctly grouped than the endocervical counterpart.

Cells of large, nonkeratinizing squamous cancer may be extremely difficult to differentiate from some endocervical, but seldom endometrial, adenocarcinomas. Individual cells of large, nonkeratinizing squamous cancer and cervical adenocarcinoma may display similar nuclear and cytoplasmic characteristics, i.e., they have prominent nucleoli, clumped nuclear chromatin and similar cytoplasmic features. Large, nonkeratinizing squamous cancer may be distinguished on smears by the frequency of syncytial cell groupings with markedly irregular borders. These groupings are infrequent in endocervical adenocarcinoma. Additionally, smears from squamous cancer have a "dirty" background, while this feature is uncommon in endocervical adenocarcinoma.

At times, hyperplastic endocervical cells may be confused with cells from cervical adenocarcinoma. It is germane to recall that the large size of hyperplastic endocervical cells is not accompanied by an abnormal nuclear/cytoplasmic ratio, nor are there malignant nuclear characteristics. Both are features foreign to cervical adenocarcinoma. Large cell size alone is not necessarily a feature of malignancy, as is pointed out in Chapter 20. Cells in smears from endocervical hypertrophy commonly appear in scattered groupings, indicative of the generally focal nature of the process. Endocervical adenocarcinoma, except for rarely occurring minimal lesions, is generally characterized by smears containing a large number of widely scattered abnormal cells.

References

1. Abell, M. R., and Gosling, J. R. G.: Gland cell carcinoma (adenocarcinoma) of the uterine cervix, Am. J. Obst. & Gynec. 83:729, 1962.
2. Buttenberg, D., and Stoll, P.: Cyto- and histomorphology of carcinoma of the Gartnerian duct, Acta cytol. 4:344, 1960.
3. Cullen, T. S.: *Cancer of the Uterus* (New York: D. Appleton & Company, 1900).
4. Davis, E. W., Jr.: Carcinoma of the corpus uteri. A study of 525 cases at New York Hospital, Am. J. Obst. & Gynec. 88:163, 1964.
5. Dougherty, C. M., and Cotton, N.: Mixed squamous-cell and adenocarcinoma of the cervix, Cancer 17:1132, 1964.
6. Friedell, G. H., and McKay, D. G.: Adenocarcinoma in situ of the endocervix, Cancer 6:887, 1953.

7. Glucksmann, A.: Histomorphology of cervical carcinoma during pregnancy (disc.), Acta cytol. 3:54, 1959.
8. Hepler, T. K., Dockerty, M. B., and Randall, L. M.: Primary adenocarcinoma of the cervix, Am. J. Obst. & Gynec. 63:800, 1952.
9. Hopman, B. C.: Cytology of endocervical adenocarcinoma, Acta cytol. 4:331, 1960.
10. Kjellgren, O.: Cytology of endocervical adenocarcinoma (disc.), Acta cytol. 4:335, 1960.
11. Krimmenau, R.: Cytology of endocervical adenocarcinoma (disc.), Acta cytol. 4:335, 1960.
12. Melnick, P. J., Lees, L. E., Jr., and Walsh, H. M.: Endocervical and cervical neoplasms adjacent to carcinoma in situ, Am. J. Clin. Path. 28:354, 1957.
13. Nuovo, V. M.: Can one distinguish by means of cytology the endocervical and endometrial adenocarcinoma? Acta cytol. 4:340, 1960.
14. Reagan, J. W., and Ng, A. B. P.: *The Cells of Uterine Adenocarcinoma* (Baltimore: Williams & Wilkins Company, 1965).
15. Sachs, O.: Die Entwickelung der Carcinome. Diss. inaug. Breslau, 1869, 8, quoted by Waldeyer.
16. Steiner, G., and Friedell, G. H.: Adenosquamous carcinoma in situ of the cervix, Cancer 18:807, 1965.
17. Tweeddale, D. N., Early, L. S., and Goodsitt, E. S.: Endometrial adenoacanthoma. A clinical and pathologic analysis of 82 cases with observations on histogenesis, Obst. & Gynec. 23:611, 1964.
18. Tweeddale, D. N., et al.: Cervical vs. endometrial carcinoma, Obst. & Gynec. 2:623, 1953.
19. von Haam, E.: Cytology of endocervical adenocarcinoma, (disc.), Acta cytol. 4:335, 1960.
20. Waldeyer, H. W.: Die Entwickelung der Carcinome, Virchows Arch. path. Anat. 55:67, 1872.

CHAPTER 14

Uterine Corpus: Anatomic and Cytologic Considerations

Gross Description

IN THE HUMAN, the upper portion of the uterus is called the corpus uteri; the pear-shaped segment is delineated at its lower limit by the internal cervical os and at its uppermost limit by the fundus uteri. The corpus in its normal state is flattened in a dorsoventral direction so that the inner surfaces of the uterine cavity are apposed to form a slit-like triangular space. The form, shape and position of the uterus vary at different periods of life and under different circumstances. In the fetus and infant, the normal fundus protrudes above the pelvic inlet, while at puberty it lies below that level. The position of the nondiseased uterus in the adult varies with both the individual's posture and the size and content of the bladder and rectum. When both are empty and the individual is in a standing position, the corpus is nearly horizontal. In that position, the fundus is only about 2 cm. behind the symphysis pubis; the uterus and vagina are at about a 90° angle with each other. In old age, the corpus usually atrophies and a more distinct constriction may appear between the uterine body and the cervix, at times so extreme as to obliterate the internal os.

The corpus uteri is divided into three layers: an outer layer, consisting of a serous membrane, or peritoneum, which incompletely covers the surface; a middle layer, consisting of a variably thick, smooth muscle coat (myometrium); and an inner layer of mucous membrane (endometrium).[5]

The cytologist is concerned primarily with changes that occur in the mucous membrane. The mucosa is smooth, soft and pale red; its thickness depends on numerous factors, of which the most important is the hormonal state of the individual.

Microscopic Considerations

Histologically, the endometrium consists of a surface layer of simple columnar epithelium which in some places is ciliated. The surface epi-

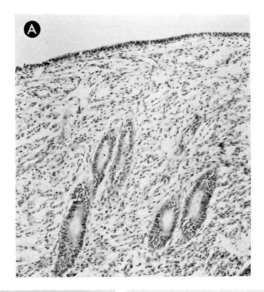

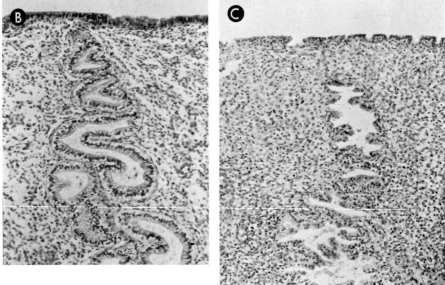

Fig. 14-1. — Endometrial changes during the normal monthly menstrual cycle. **A,** early proliferative phase. Cells which form the straight glands contain numerous mitotic figures, as do the cells of the accompanying stroma. **B,** early secretory phase showing glands that are more tortuous. Stromal cells are still small and round and mitotic figures are absent. Subnuclear secretory vacuoles are present in most cells. **C,** late secretory phase evidencing even greater tortuosity of glands. Secretory vacuoles have disappeared because the secretion has been discharged into the gland lumens; consequently, lining cells are more irregular and flatter than those observed in earlier secretory stages. Stromal cells in the upper and middle layers of the endometrium have increased in size due to increased cytoplasmic mass. Mitotic figures are absent.

thelium is continuous with columnar epithelium that forms intramucosal glands, which extend through the entire thickness of the mucosa. The epithelium is supported by stroma resembling mesenchyme, as the constituent cells are irregularly stellate and have poorly demarcated cytoplasm. The stroma varies in cellularity and the cells differ morphologically at different levels of the endometrium and with different phases of the menstrual cycle. The stromal vasculature varies similarly with the cycle; scattered lymphocytes and macrophages may be present at certain times in variable numbers.

In order to better understand normal cytologic findings, it is necessary to review the endometrial changes that occur during the normal monthly menstrual cycle, designed to prepare the mucosa for reception of the fertilized ovum.[11]

The proliferative or follicular phase is between the 5th and the 14th day of a normal 28-day cycle; typically, it is associated with a rapidly growing, estrogen-producing Graafian follicle. At the beginning of this period, the endometrium is thin and flat, the surface and in continuity glandular epithelium being cuboidal to low columnar. The glands have small lumens, are sparse and short. The compact stroma is composed of small, poorly demarcated cells (Fig. 14-1, A). Epithelial and stromal cells both show mitotic activity. Later in this phase, several different surface cell types are clearly recognizable. Most are simple columnar cells, while those that are ciliated and intercalated are present in lesser numbers. As the cycle progresses, the glands become more numerous, more closely approximated and more tortuous; the lining epithelium becomes tall columnar with pseudostratified nuclei. Similarly, the stromal cells also proliferate and enlarge. Mitotic activity is quite conspicuous in both epithelium and stroma.

After ovulation, there is usually a lapse of 2 days before the endometrium changes into its secretory or luteal phase, characterized by the appearance of secretory products in glandular cells and a cessation of mitotic activity (Fig. 14-1, B). This phase reflects the formation of an ovarian corpus luteum which secretes progesterone. The mucosa is thicker and slightly more irregular than in the proliferative phase of the cycle and is covered by tall columnar epithelium. The glands become denser, more tortuous and have wider lumens than those in the first half of the cycle. On the 17th day, the glandular epithelium contains a subnuclear vacuole that displaces the nucleus upwards to a more central position. Within a 24-hour period, this vacuole slips past the nucleus to assume a supranuclear location, displacing the nucleus downward so that it is once again positioned at the base of the cell. Shortly thereafter, the secretory product (a glycoprotein) is extruded from the cell and is apparent in the lumens of endometrial glands.

On about the 21st day, stromal cells become edematous and enlarge.

Simultaneously, both the glands and glandular epithelium undergo involution. The stromal cells, on about the 27th day, enlarge further, especially around arterioles in the upper portion of the endometrium (Fig. 14-1, C).

Just preceding menstruation, vascular compromise leads to ischemia, focal necrosis and endometrial hemorrhage, especially in the upper two thirds of the endometrium. The entire endometrium sheds over a 3–5 day period, except for the basal portion (basalis) from which the endometrium regenerates to start the proliferative phase of the cycle. The regenerative process is so rapid that the surface epithelium may be restored completely by the 4th day of the next 28-day cycle.[8]

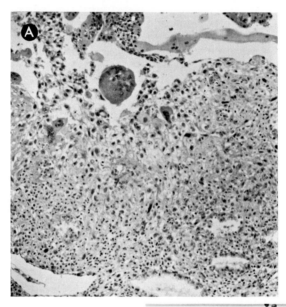

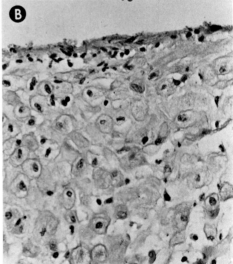

Fig. 14-2. — Appearance of the endometrium during pregnancy. **A,** histologic section from a woman who was one-month pregnant. A primitive trophoblast can be seen in the upper part of the section. Stromal cells are larger and glands less conspicuous than in sections taken from non-pregnant females (Fig. 14-1). **B,** decidual cells in a histologic section from a woman in mid-pregnancy. These cells are considerably larger than in **A** and the nuclei are often large with prominent nucleoli. The nuclear/cytoplasmic ratio does not suggest malignancy, however.

The endometrium varies in microscopic appearance with the patient's gestational status and age. Early pregnancy is characterized by a continuance and accentuation of the progestational stage; the glands very rapidly become even more hypertrophic and tortuous than they were during the secretory phase. The glandular epithelium is low columnar, pale and actively secretory. At a later stage, the epithelium becomes very flat, especially in cells comprising the superficial zone. The well vascularized superficial stroma is composed of large, polygonal cells with clearly demarcated, copious granular cytoplasm, central nuclei and prominent nucleoli (stromal cells throughout gestation are called decidual cells) (Fig. 14-2, A). Cell membranes are coated with a thin layer of amorphous material, with the histochemical characteristics of a mucopolysaccharide. At the height of their development, the stromal cells range in size from 30–100 microns in diameter and it is not unusual for some of the larger cells to be multinucleated (Fig. 14-2, B). In general, stromal cells decrease in size during the third trimester. By contrast, stromal cells forming the basalis retain their nonprogestational and nondecidual character. It is also pertinent that this endometrial pattern may reflect an extrauterine pregnancy.

Because of more extensive denudation of the uterine lining following delivery, postpartum regeneration is a slower process than postmenstrual repair. Oozing of blood or blood-tinged serum ("lochia") may be expected to continue for up to 4 weeks; at times, because of delayed regeneration, months may pass before menstruation resumes, even though ovulation has commenced.[9]

In the newborn, the endometrium may show some secretory glandu-

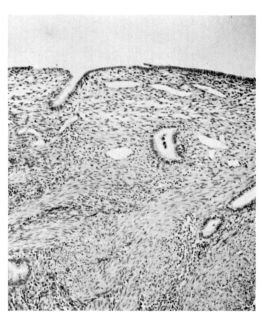

Fig. 14-3. — Histologic section from a postmenopausal woman with atrophic endometrium. Glands and stroma forming the thin endometrium are atrophic. At times, however, these women may have hypertrophied glandular epithelium without an altered nuclear/cytoplasmic ratio. Ciliated cells may be commonly encountered but in cytologic smears cilia are observed only by careful study.

lar activity and patches of stromal decidual change due to transplacental transfer of circulating maternal hormones. In infancy and early childhood, the endometrium is characteristically thin, with widely scattered glands surrounded by a stroma that is compact, dense and somewhat fibrous. Immediately before menarche, the increase in circulating estrogens so stimulates the endometrium that it resembles that of the early proliferative phase. In the postmenopausal period, the endometrium is usually atrophic (Fig. 14-3). The stromal cells are small, spindled and angular, dense and fibrous appearing. Both surface and glandular epithelium are cuboidal or flat and are generally devoid of mitotic activity.[4]

Cytologic Considerations

It is apparent that the cells that constitute normal endometrium vary predictably with age as well as with the phases of the menstrual cycle. Obviously, before an understanding of the abnormal can be achieved, the cytologist must acquire mastery of the many nuances of morphology that may normally be encountered in the cells lining the uterine cavity.

The method by which the specimen was obtained (i.e., forcible aspiration or spontaneous desquamation) may affect cellular morphology. In general, the cytologic characteristics of cells obtained by the former technique tend to resemble closely those of the same cells in situ (Fig. 14-4, A). The epithelial cells are prismatic and are often arranged in groupings similar to those of the cells in situ. However, cells obtained following spontaneous desquamation are affected by the fluid environment into which they are shed. Consequently, whether encountered singly or in groups, they tend to become more spherical (Fig. 14-4, B). If they have been so detached for a significant period of time, they may undergo degenerative changes.

The number of endometrial cells also varies with the type of specimen collection. With a properly performed endometrial aspiration, endometrial cells are regularly seen in most, if not all, specimens regardless of the phase of the cycle. Between menarche and menopause, in specimens that depend on spontaneous desquamation, however, endometrial cells are normally found in steadily decreasing numbers between the first and fifteenth days of the cycle (Fig. 14-5). They are rarely seen in the second half of the cycle. Indeed, the mere presence of these cells in a phase of the cycle in which they are not normally expected should be viewed with suspicion. Endometrial cells are so rarely seen in smears from postmenopausal women that their presence should always be viewed with suspicion and ignite a search for an underlying pathologic process.[10]

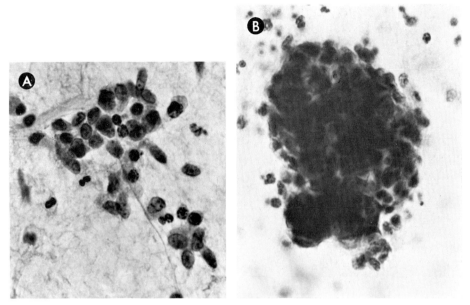

Fig. 14-4. – Comparison of cells of the normal endometrium. **A,** cells obtained by forcible aspiration appear singly and grouped. They are small and columnar shaped which implies recent exfoliation. Following exfoliation they tend to assume a round shape. The nucleus occupies less than 50% of the total cell area and the cytoplasm is light cyanophilic. The round nucleus may be in different locations in the cells, i.e., from base to lumen, depending on the stage of the endometrial cycle. Nuclear chromatin is finely dispersed and a single, small nucleolus can be seen with difficulty. **B,** a fairly large group of clustered cells for a menstruating woman (spontaneous desquamation). They are very small, tightly packed and show clumped nuclear chromatin, probably a degenerative phenomenon. Cytoplasmic outlines are often indistinct. Polymorphonuclear leukocytes and erythrocytes can be seen in the background. These small, partially degenerated, endometrial cells should not be misdiagnosed to represent cancer. Cytologic findings can usually be supported by historic data.

DISTRIBUTION OF ENDOMETRIAL CELLS

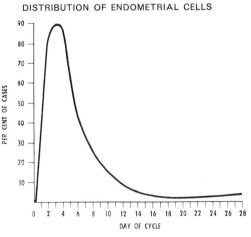

Fig. 14-5. – Occurrence of endometrial cells in aspirates from the cervical canal in relation to day of menstrual cycle. (From Reagan, J. W., and Ng., A. B. P.: *The Cells of Uterine Adenocarcinoma* [Baltimore: Williams and Wilkins Company, 1965].)

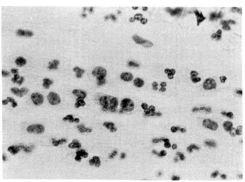

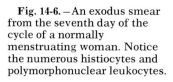

Fig. 14-6. – An exodus smear from the seventh day of the cycle of a normally menstruating woman. Notice the numerous histiocytes and polymorphonuclear leukocytes.

Desquamated endometrial cells may be present following abortion or in the immediate postpartum period for variable periods of time; in these situations, they are seldom of malignant nature.

Elements derived from non-neoplastic endometrial lining that can be identified in cytologic smears include epithelial cells that are secretory, ciliated and intercalated, as well as endometrial stromal cells, fibrin, erythrocytes and a variety of inflammatory cells (Fig. 14-6). The following section includes a description of formed elements that may be encountered in specimens from the endometrium, either directly or following spontaneous exfoliation.

Specific Cytologic Characteristics of Cells from the Endometrium

The epithelial cells of the endometrium are shed in groups or, less commonly, singly. Groupings may consist solely of epithelial cells or epithelial cells in combination with stromal cells. The exfoliated groups often form dense balls of cells rendering fine nuclear detail difficult to delineate (Fig. 14-4). Some groups evidently consist of a peripheral rim of epithelial cells surrounding a central core of stromal cells.

Secretory nonciliated cells. – The secretory, nonciliated cell is the endometrial cell most commonly observed in cytologic specimens. The spontaneously desquamated, isolated cells are small and round or oval. The usually eccentric nuclei have a mean area of 30.6 ± 4.5 square microns and are also round or oval. Nuclear chromatin is evenly distributed and finely granular; nucleoli are rarely identified. The cytoplasm is scant and ill defined, especially in the proliferative phase, but enlarges in the secretory phase. Cytoplasmic staining characteristics are variable; one or more vacuoles may be apparent. In the postmenopausal period, endometrial cells may be smaller than those seen during the reproductive years. If for any reason epithelial cells are derived from the basalis, they will resemble those in the proliferative phase regardless of the menstrual phase.

In endometrial aspiration specimens, the cell clusters are more sharply delineated with definite glandular structures identifiable. The epithelial cells are more angular and, with proper orientation, can be identified as columnar. The height of these cells tends to increase during the menstrual cycle, but the round or oval nucleus does not change in size throughout the cycle. The chromatin pattern is indistinct in the early part of the proliferative phase, but subsequently becomes distinctly granular. The cytoplasm is initially basophilic, but it becomes amphophilic or eosinophilic during the secretory phase when there are also variably located vacuoles. In some cells, the vacuoles impinge on the nucleus and distort its contour.[10] The average nuclear area throughout the proliferative and secretory phases of the cycle is 40 μ^2; the nuclear diameter is 6–10 μ.[6]

INTERCALATED CELLS. – These cells are of similar size to the secretory cell and probably represent compressed secretory cells. After exfoliation, they become spherical and are indistinguishable from the secretory cell. In endometrial aspiration specimens with optimal orientation, they are long and slender with a central bulge related to the nucleus.[10]

CILIATED EPITHELIAL CELLS. – Even though ciliated epithelium is abundant in cyclical endometrium, cilia are not easily recognizable in exfoliated material. By contrast, in aspiration specimens, cilia may be observed readily in columnar cells with basal nuclei.[3]

ENDOMETRIAL STROMAL CELLS. – The stromal cells from different levels of the endometrium vary in appearance. These cells are shed singly or in groups, and the latter may be indistinguishable from clusters of epithelial cells. Isolated cells have a finely vacuolated, poorly stained and ill-defined cytoplasm. The nuclei are round, oval, spindled or reniform. In the early proliferative phase, the chromatin is finely granular but becomes more coarsely granular as the phase progresses. In the secretory phase, the chromatin appears more compact. Cells desquamated during the proliferative phase, or from the basalis, are small with an oval or spindle-shaped nucleus and have a small amount of minimally vacuolated cytoplasm. During the secretory period, the stromal cells originating from the upper endometrial zone increase almost twofold in size. A smear containing both populations of stromal cells suggests that there has been a progesterone response and that, in addition, the endometrium has been shed to expose deeper layers. In the late secretory phase, variable phagocytosis may be observed.

In endometrial aspirates, variations in appearance of stromal cells during different parts of the cycle are more easily seen. There is progressive enlargement of these cells from 45 square microns on the 7th day of the cycle to 72 square microns on the 13th day. From that time until the 18th to the 20th day of the cycle, the cells enlarge further to reach the maximal size, which persists until menstruation. The nuclear and cytoplasmic characteristics of the cells are similar to those in exfoliated specimens. In the latter part of the cycle, there is a gradual transition towards an appearance reminiscent of histiocytes, and, indeed, such cells may be actively phagocytic. There tends, in general, to be a greater variation in nuclear size in clusters of stromal cells than in clusters of glandular cells, especially when observed in the secretory phase.[1,2,6] The suggestive syncytial appearance of the clusters during the proliferative phase helps in identifying these cells, even though they may appear hyperchromatic.[6]

During the postmenopausal period, aspiration specimens almost always yield cells. Some smears show a typical proliferative type of epithelium and stroma; others show elongated cells with slight anisokaryosis and hyperchromasia, or isokaryotic cells which are more hypochromatic and smaller than those from menstruating women.[6]

REFERENCES

1. Boschann, H. W.: Cytomorphology of normal endometrium, Acta cytol. 2:505, 1958.
2. Boschann, H. W.: Cytometry on normal and abnormal endometrial cells, Acta cytol. 2: 520, 1958.
3. Flemming, S., Tweeddale, D. N., and Roddick, J. W., Jr.: Ciliated endometrial cells, Am. J. Obst. & Gynec. 102:186, 1968.
4. Goldecht, J. J.: *Gynecological Endocrinology* (New York: Paul B. Hoeber, Inc., 1968), p. 193.
5. Goss, C. M. (ed.): *Gray's Anatomy of the Human Body* (26th ed.; Philadelphia: Lea & Febiger, 1954), pp. 1348–1403.
6. Horava, A., *et al.*: The exfoliative cytologic characteristics of the endometrium and health and disease, Clin. Obst. & Gynec. 4:1128, 1961.
7. Nieburgs, H. E.: Histiocytes and endometrial cytology, Acta cytol. 2:518, 1958.
8. Noyes, R. W., and Hertig, A.: Dating the endometrium, Fertil. and Steril. 1:1, 1950.
9. Patten, B. M.: *Human Embryology* (3d. ed.; New York: McGraw-Hill Book Company, Inc., 1968), pp. 124–130.
10. Reagan, J. W., and Ng, A. B. P.: *The Cells of Uterine Adenocarcinoma* (Baltimore: Williams and Wilkins Company, 1965).
11. Schmidt-Mathiesen, H. (ed.): *The Normal Human Endometrium* (New York: McGraw-Hill Book Company, Inc., 1963).

CHAPTER 15

The Cytopathology of Endometrial Adenocarcinoma

Introduction

THE CYTODIAGNOSTIC accuracy of endometrial carcinoma is less than that of cervical malignancy. Utilizing cervicovaginal smears obtained under usual screening conditions, different observers have been able to identify either malignant or suspicious cells in 50% – 94% of women with endometrial cancer. Using vaginal cytology, we were able to demonstrate such cells in 64.3% of 28 proven cases of primary endometrial adenocarcinoma. Endometrial aspiration preparations, in consort with routine vaginal smears, greatly enhance the accuracy of cytodiagnosis of endometrial cancer.[4, 12, 13, 25, 30, 31, 38, 40, 42] The success of aspiration techniques confirms the dictum that cytologic material should be collected in closest possible proximity to a suspected lesion. However, the practicality of endometrial aspiration as a routine screening procedure, even in postmenopausal women, is highly controversial.[4, 17] The following sections briefly discuss the clinical and histologic features of endometrial cancer. Detailed cellular characteristics in smear preparations, either following aspiration or spontaneous exfoliation, are presented. In general, the findings in our cases are similar to those of other investigators.

Clinical Correlates

Endometrial carcinoma is a disease characteristically observed in postmenopausal women; in fact, only about 2% – 5% of females with that condition are less than 40 years of age.[11, 20, 36] All of our patients were older than 40 and only 2 were less than 50 years of age. About 40% of patients with cancer of the upper uterine segment are nulligravidas, sharply contrasting with the consistently observed multiparity of women with cervical squamous cancer. Certain clinical conditions, such as infertility, obesity, hypertension and abnormal carbohydrate

171

metabolism, frequently coexist with endometrial cancer. This association suggests that aberrant endocrine metabolism might, in some way, be partially responsible for adenocarcinoma of the endometrium.[11] Such an assumption is questionably valid; these clinical conditions may be encountered with equal frequency in women with either cervical or endometrial cancer, provided they are age matched.[32]

The ratio of endometrial adenocarcinoma to cervical squamous cancer is dependent on the socioeconomic structure of the patient population. For example, among patients seen in private office practice, the ratio may be at least 1:1, while in a charity clinic population the ratio may be 1 endometrial to greater than 20 cervical cancers. The earlier average age of coitus and, to a lesser degree, increased parity among those from a socioeconomically depressed group, probably account for the relatively higher incidence of cervical cancer among them.[36]

Gross Morphologic Aspects of Endometrial Cancer

Endometrial adenocarcinoma has a greater tendency to arise in the upper portion of the endometrium, but no endometrial area is immune. The neoplasm is first seen as a small, flat, circumscribed lesion, although, at times, it apparently originates from a more diffuse area of a variably thickened endometrial lining. By progressive growth the tumor eventually enlarges to form either a polypoid or, less frequently, a broad-based and lobulated lesion. Spread to the myometrium or adjacent endometrium may occur at any time. The tumors are likely to be friable with variable-sized areas of necrosis and/or hemorrhage, accounting for the spontaneous exfoliation of malignant cells as well as the "diathesis" (see Fig. 15-3) seen in cytosmears. Adjacent uninvolved endometrium may appear normal, atrophic or hyperplastic and seldom sheds cells in numbers approaching those shed by cancerous areas.[11, 20]

Histologic Features of Adenocarcinoma of the Corpus Uteri

Application of cytology to the diagnosis of endometrial cancer depends on knowledge of the many and varied changes within the neoplasm and the adjacent tissue. A thorough understanding of non-neoplastic cellular reactions of the endometrium resulting from different types of injury or stimuli is necessary to avoid diagnostic errors. Also, the subtle histologic transitions from hyperplasia to carcinoma in situ and adenocarcinoma must be recognized in order to better understand the smear findings. Graphically, this morphologic gradation can be illustrated by the following scheme, representing lesions of increasing severity: cystic hyperplasia→ glandular hyperplasia→ adenomatous hyperplasia→ adenocarcinoma in situ→ invasive adenocarcinoma. The relationship of endometrial hyperplasia to carcinoma is a statistical

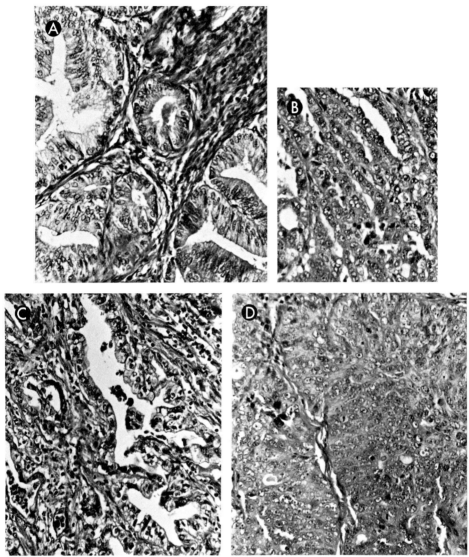

Fig. 15-1. – Uterine adenocarcinoma. **A,** histologic pattern of a well-differentiated grade I uterine carcinoma. Diagnosis is based primarily on the back-to-back arrangement of the glands. Neither nuclear hyperchromasia, nuclear enlargement or alteration in the nuclear/cytoplasmic ratio shows significant deviation from that encountered in hyperplasia. Reduced from ×64. **B** and **C,** grade II. The cells are smaller and more closely packed than in grade I lesions. The nuclei show greater pleomorphism and contain prominent single nucleoli. Reduced from ×64. **D,** poorly differentiated grade III adenocarcinoma of the uterus. Gland spaces are difficult to identify and mitotic figures are common. Nuclei contain various-sized prominent nucleoli. Reduced from ×64.

one, since only a minority of hyperplasias progress to invasive cancer. Unfortunately, at present there is no means of distinguishing between hyperplasias that will and those that will not progress to cancer.

In general, most cases of cystic and glandular hyperplasia can be easily recognized in histologic sections. By contrast, differentiation between severe adenomatous hyperplasia and carcinoma in situ may present problems in tissue diagnosis and, unfortunately, that difficulty is also reflected in cytologic material. Like other malignant neoplasms, those of endometrial origin can be subdivided according to degree of histologic differentiation (Fig. 15-1): well differentiated → moderately well differentiated → poorly differentiated → undifferentiated. Cancers closely resembling normal endometrial glands are well differentiated. With increasing aberration from the normal gland structure, the neoplasms are classified as poorly differentiated, and, in some cases, the dedifferentiation is so great that painstaking study is necessary to identify them as adenocarcinoma.

As indicated, diagnostic difficulties in tissue sections have their counterparts in cytologic preparations so that it may not be possible to distinguish cytologically among some cases of hyperplasia, carcinoma in situ and low-grade invasive cancer. Of 10 histologically proven cases with endometrial carcinoma that were cytologically negative for malignancy, 8 were grade I tumors. When tissue findings are those of a more poorly differentiated neoplasm, positive cytologic smears will almost always be encountered. In most endometrial cancer cases, the cytologic

Fig. 15-2. – Histologic section of a mucin-producing uterine adenocarcinoma, grade II. ×64.

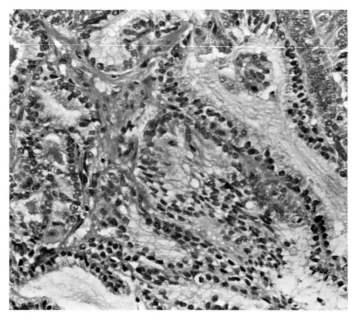

material will create sufficient suspicion, either by background or cellular findings, as to suggest the requirement for histologic study.

In addition to glandular and epithelial changes in endometrial adenocarcinoma, one frequently encounters surface ulceration, necrosis, hemorrhage and inflammation. Rarely, tumor cells may produce mucus, resulting in a blood-stained mucoid vaginal discharge (Fig. 15-2). In some cases, especially in well-differentiated cancers, there may be stromal collections of foamy histiocytes reflecting the phagocytosis of lipid material released from necrotic cells.[18, 22, 35]

A frequent variant of adenocarcinoma of the endometrium is the adenoacanthoma pattern. Histologically, this appears as an adenocarcinoma, usually low grade, within which there is a variable metaplastic change, usually to benign squamous epithelium.[35] Those endometrial carcinomas in which the squamous elements are also malignant have a decidedly poorer prognosis.[27]

Cytologic Features of Adenocarcinoma of the Corpus Uteri

NON-NEOPLASTIC SMEAR FINDINGS. — Smear analysis is initiated by systematic scanning of slides under low magnification, not only to identify obvious neoplastic cells, but to assess certain non-neoplastic findings that may be associated with cancer.

Such non-neoplastic smear findings from patients with endometrial adenocarcinoma include various combinations of red blood cells, cellular exudate, fibrin and cellular debris—the so-called "diathesis" (Fig. 15-3, A). The importance of this finding is emphasized by studies of Reagan and Ng who encountered it in 90% of well-differentiated cancers and 100% of the poorly differentiated ones. Large histiocytes were present in about 28% of all their tumors (Fig. 15-3, B). Some investigators have maintained that there is evidence of increased estrogenic effect in smears from patients with endometrial cancer in the form of a greater number of karyopyknotic vaginal cells.[14, 41] That view, however, is controversial, since others have found cytohormonal patterns from such patients to be comparable with normal postmenopausal women.[5, 31, 42]

ENDOMETRIAL CELLS IN SMEARS. — The cytologic diagnosis of cancer is ultimately based on the qualitative characteristics of the cells present. In certain instances, however, the mere presence of endometrial cells in vaginal pool smears is abnormal and warrants further investigation. For example, in premenopausal women, the presence of such cells is considered abnormal only after the first 15 days of the menstrual period[31]; in fact, Liu, et al.,[24] found that only 1% of females revealed endometrial cells in smears after 10 days. On the other hand, in postmenopausal women, the group in which most endometrial cancers

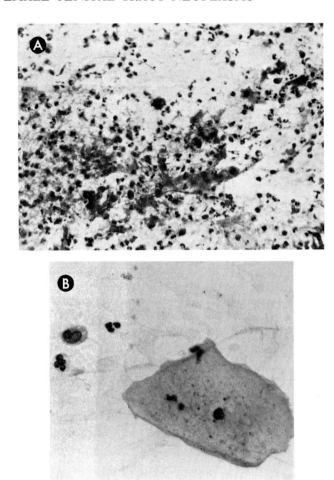

Fig. 15-3.—Non-neoplastic smear findings from patients with uterine adenocarcinoma. **A,** smear demonstrating the "diathesis" with inflammatory exudate, characterized by debris, fibrin and scattered histiocytes—findings often associated with endometrial carcinoma. ×64. **B,** smear showing a karyopyknotic superficial squamous cell, a histiocyte and scattered polymorphonuclear leukocytes. The histiocyte may be difficult to differentiate from an endometrial glandular or stromal cell. Compare with Figure 15-4C. ×160.

occur, the mere presence of endometrial cells in smears is considered to be an abnormal finding.

Characteristics of Malignant Cells Seen in Endometrial Adenocarcinoma

GENERAL CELL CHARACTERISTICS (Fig. 15-4). — Tumor cells in smears may appear isolated or in clusters.[15] Tumors with a papillary appearance in histologic material tend to shed more cells, both isolated and in clusters, than tumors that are not papillary. The clusters can vary in size from small, compact, rounded cell masses to large, rounded or irregular cell groupings. Groupings tend to be more common in less differentiated lesions.[31] All but one of our cytologically diagnosable smears contained cell clusters.

CELL SIZE. — In general, the desquamated cells of endometrial carcinomas are significantly larger than normal endometrial cells. In one study, the mean area of the tumor cells was 148.7 ± 53.1 square microns (1 standard deviation).[31] The large standard deviation supports the observation that cells in smears from endometrial cancer vary greatly in size; it further suggests that in a single sample, a significant proportion of the cancer cells may approach the normal endometrial cells in size. Tumor cells increase in size in direct proportion to increasing histologic grade of malignancy. For example, the mean cell area of well-differentiated tumors is 132.0 μ^2 ± 48.3 μ^2, with progressive increase in area to 198.1 ± 79.8 μ^2 for poorly differentiated neoplasms.[31]

CELL CONFIGURATION. — Desquamated and isolated cells in vaginal cytologic specimens assume round or oval shapes, reflecting effects of residence in the vaginal pool on the cells that were originally columnar. When they are present in groups, it is often difficult to determine the shape of individual cells.

NUCLEAR SIZE AND SHAPE. — Spontaneously desquamated cells rarely have more than a single nucleus. The nucleus is characteristically eccentric and is either oval or round. Nuclei are seldom irregular in shape, except when distorted by cytoplasmic vacuoles. As determined by planimetry, the mean nuclear area of these cancer cells is 68.0 ± 17.2 μ^2, while that of normal endometrial cells is 30.6 ± 4.5 μ^2.[31] In general, the mean nuclear size of normal cells in endometrial aspirates is about 33% greater than those in vaginal specimens.[31] A gradual increase in mean nuclear area (60 to 91.7 μ^2) and also a greater variation in nuclear size is associated with increasing grade of malignancy.[31]

NUCLEAR/CYTOPLASMIC RATIO. — Nuclei of endometrial cancer cells generally occupy a larger proportion of the mean cellular area than normal. Reagan and Ng[31] report that cells from all grades of adenocarcinoma contained nuclei averaging 44% to 48% of the total cell area.

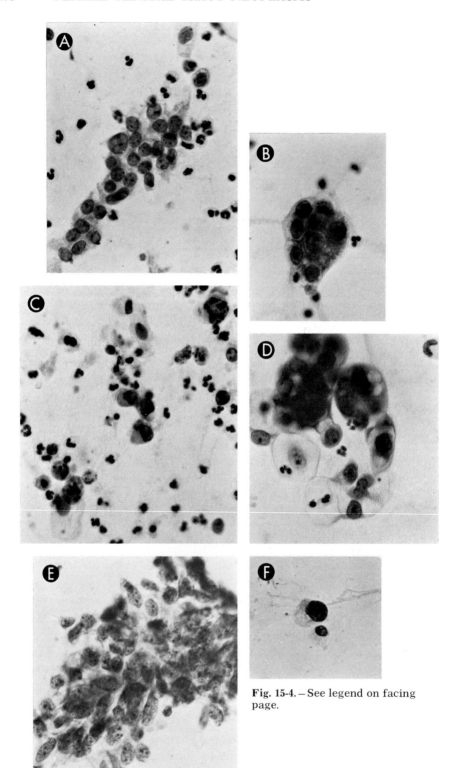

Fig. 15-4. — See legend on facing page.

Most of our cases had a nucleus that occupied about half the cell area. The presence of large cytoplasmic vacuoles, which may appear following desquamation, may so alter the nuclear/cytoplasmic ratio that it falls within the normal range. It is also worthy to note that in a single case there may be a significant variation in nuclear/cytoplasmic ratio in cells that show relatively little over-all size variation.

CHROMATIN PATTERN AND NUCLEAR MEMBRANE. – The majority of adenocarcinoma cells in smear preparations have a well-defined, thin nuclear membrane. In a small number of cells, the nuclear membrane may be thickened by an underlying accumulation of chromatin. Otherwise, nuclear chromatin is irregularly distributed and is usually finely granular. In general, the nuclei of most cells, even from tumors of high histologic grade, are only slightly hyperchromatic.[31] Since hyperchromasia is generally proportionate to nuclear DNA, it is of interest that the DNA content in 80% of endometrial carcinomas is consistent with a diploid number of chromosomes.[3] These characteristics are particularly useful in distinguishing them from the cells of cervical adenocarcinoma, which frequently show aneuploidy.

NUCLEOLI. – Unlike normal endometrial cells, whose nucleoli are barely visible, almost 90% of adenocarcinoma cells have visible nucleoli, usually single and of variable size. About one third of cells contain more than one nucleolus. Larger and multiple nucleoli tend to be more commonly observed in less differentiated neoplasms. In general, the majority of nucleoli are round and regular, except in the most poorly differentiated tumors.[31]

CYTOPLASMIC COLOR AND CONTENT. – The cytoplasmic color of endometrial adenocarcinoma cells, using the Papanicolaou stain, may be cyanophilic, eosinophilic or amphophilic. Such variability in staining precludes the use of tinctorial characteristics to identify the specific

←

Fig. 15-4. – Uterine adenocarcinoma smears from spontaneously exfoliated material. **A**, smear from the grade I tumor shown in Figure 15-1A demonstrating a cluster of desquamated cells with round, slightly enlarged and hyperchromatic nuclei. The nuclei vary slightly in size and have a small but distinct nucleolus. Reduced from ×160. **B**, smear from the grade II tumor in Figure 15-1B showing a rounded cluster of desquamated neoplastic cells. The round nuclei are larger than those found in grade I endometrial adenocarcinoma, are moderately hyperchromatic, slightly eccentric and contain prominent nucleoli. The nucleus occupies a greater per cent of the total cell area than in grade I adenocarcinoma. Reduced from ×160. **C**, smear from the grade II tumor shown in Figure 15-1C demonstrating isolated desquamated neoplastic cells. The cytologic findings are similar to those in **B** except for greater nuclear irregularity. Reduced from ×160. **D**, smear from the grade II tumor illustrated in Figure 15-2 showing a cluster of desquamated neoplastic cells with a slightly hyperchromic nuclei, prominent nucleoli and fairly abundant, clear, markedly vacuolated cytoplasm. Reduced from ×160. **E**, smear from the tumor shown in Figure 15-1D demonstrating an irregular cluster of desquamated neoplastic cells with generally ovoid irregular nuclei containing coarse chromatin and prominent nucleoli. Size variability between individual nuclei is evident and cytoplasmic borders are indistinct. Reduced from ×160. **F**, another smear from the tumor illustrated in 15-1D which shows an isolated neoplastic cell with an eccentric, very hyperchromatic nucleus and no discernible nucleolus. Reduced from ×160.

character of desquamated cells. The cytoplasm may appear homogeneous, granular or contain diffusely distributed fine vacuoles. Large, discrete vacuoles are seen in less than one fifth of all cases and decrease in frequency with diminishing differentiation.[31]

ADENOACANTHOMA. — Most cells desquamated from endometrial adenoacanthomas are comparable to those of the usual endometrial adenocarcinoma. The squamous component is not uniformly desquamated and, of course, may not be recognizable as malignant. Diagnosis of an endometrial adenoacanthoma is only feasible when a group of neoplastic adenocarcinoma cells is intimately associated with benign squamous elements. When neoplastic glandular elements are associated with malignant squamous cells, it is difficult to ascertain whether they represent two separate tumors or an adenoacanthoma with a malignant squamous component.

Differential Cytodiagnosis of Endometrial Adenocarcinoma

It has been established previously that the cytologic diagnosis of endometrial carcinoma frequently poses difficulties. This section emphasizes various endometrial changes that present problems in their distinction from cancer of the upper uterine segment. Noncancerous endometrial reactions, as in other tissues of the body, can be broadly classified into the following categories: atrophy, hypertrophy, hyperplasia, degeneration, necrosis, inflammation and benign neoplasia. Within this group, attention will be directed only to those conditions presenting significant diagnostic problems.

HYPERPLASIA

Hyperplasia is an abnormal, potentially reversible, growth response characterized by an increase in the number of cells normally observed in a given tissue or organ. Individual cells may exhibit qualitative changes, such as increase in size (hypertrophy), or differences in physiochemical structure. Some relate the endometrial changes to excessive, unopposed estrogen stimulation and/or an unusual receptivity of the glands and/or stroma. This abnormality may develop in either premenopausal or postmenopausal women. The endometrium shows a variable gross picture and is represented either by diffuse or polypoid thickening or, less commonly, an essentially normal appearance. The histologic appearance shows a multiplicity of patterns which obviously cannot be considered in great detail. The two most significant patterns, glandular hyperplasia and adenomatous hyperplasia, will be considered briefly. Glandular hyperplasia, with or without cystic dilatation, is characterized by an increased number of glands arranged in a disorganized pattern. The glands are usually lined by enlarged epithelial cells with

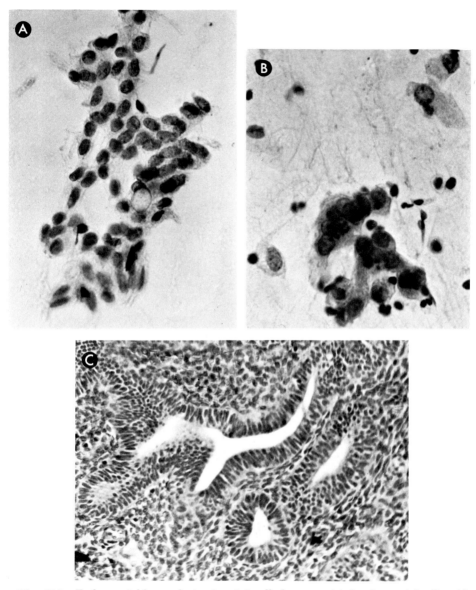

Fig. 15-5.—Endometrial hyperplasia. **A,** minimally hypertrophied endometrial cells with nuclei slightly larger than those of normal endometrial cells. Although not shown in this field, many endometrial cells from this patient had cilia. The histologic pattern varied from mild to moderate endometrial hyperplasia. **B,** large endometrial cells of endometrial hyperplasia which usually appear singly or in small groupings. The enlarged nuclei may contain fairly prominent nucleoli. At times these cells may be almost impossible to differentiate from those of low-grade endometrial adenocarcinoma. **C,** curettement specimen from the patient whose cells are shown in **B** and evidencing moderate endometrial hyperplasia.

proportionately enlarged nuclei. Evidence of intracellular or intraglandular secretory activity is most unusual. Adenomatous hyperplasia shows a greater disorganization and increase in the number of glands than in glandular hyperplasia; in the former condition, the epithelium may form intraluminal projections. The interglandular stroma is never completely obliterated, so that the glands are not arranged in the "back-to-back" pattern of adenocarcinoma.[28]

The cytologic representation of endometrial hyperplasia is as follows[2, 9, 23]:

1. There may be estrogen effect in cytohormonal preparations from the lateral vaginal wall, evidenced by an increase in the number of kary-

Fig. 15-6. — Endometrial hyperplasia. **A,** a singly appearing, round, hypertrophied endometrial gland cell is seen in the center of this field. The nucleus occupies more cell area than in normal endometrial cells (compare with Fig. 15-5 *A* and *B*) and the nucleolus is more prominent. **B,** histologic section from the patient whose cells are shown in **A.** The cells forming the glands are distinctly hypertrophied and the diagnosis was polyploid endometrial hyperplasia.

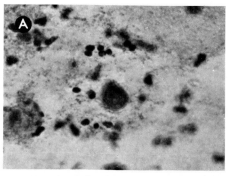

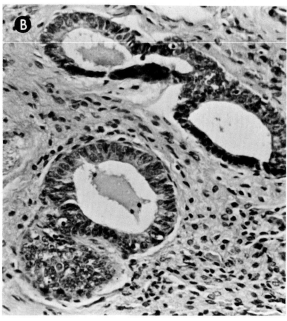

opyknotic cells, both in premenopausal and postmenopausal women.

2. There is seldom evidence of inflammatory or necrotic debris in cervicovaginal smears.

3. There are tightly packed nests of endometrial cells that closely resemble normal cells with respect to size and appearance (Fig. 15-5).

4. Single, normal-appearing endometrial epithelial cells are observed.

5. In some cases, nuclei of grouped or singly occurring cells may show uniform hyperchromasia and anisokaryosis, and contain a small nucleolus (Fig. 15-6).

The individual epithelial cells appear uniformly and remarkably similar. They have a nuclear area of 51.1 μ^2 ± 13.3 μ^2;[8] thus, their nuclei are larger than those in normal endometrial cells. At times, however, cellular findings in such instances present great diagnostic difficulties because of the overlap of the characteristics of these cells with those of low-grade endometrial cancer. Accordingly, a definitive diagnosis of endometrial hyperplasia is so seldom made on smear study alone that diagnostic curettage is mandatory. It must be strongly emphasized, however, that the mere presence of endometrial cells in postmenopausal women or in the wrong phase of the cycle in premenopausal women represents an abnormal situation requiring further investigation.

ENDOMETRIAL POLYP

A polyp is a descriptive term used to connote a localized, variably sized, rounded projection from an otherwise normal endometrial surface. These may be single or multiple, sessile or pedunculated. Uterine polyps are most commonly of endocervical origin, with those of endometrial origin second in frequency. The endometrial polyp is characterized histologically by a localized increase in glandular and/or stromal endometrial tissue, which may or may not respond to cyclical hormones secreted by the ovary. Because these polyps may show the same pathologic alterations that occur simultaneously in the endometrium (i.e., inflammation and degeneration, etc.), the cytologic manifestations are similarly protean. In general, the presence of an endometrial polyp cannot be predicted accurately by cytologic means alone. Smear findings suggestive of a benign polyp include the observation of a few tight clusters of small endometrial cells with dense nuclei composed of poorly defined chromatin and the presence of indistinct nucleoli. Compounding cytodiagnostic difficulties are the erythrocytes and inflammatory cells that are seen commonly with this lesion and, at times, a "dirty" background like that noted with endometrial adenocarcinoma.[10, 29, 33]

Cells exfoliated from submucous myomas are rarely seen in vaginal smears. At times, when these myomas enlarge or become necrotic, the already thinned overlying endometrium is compressed further and sloughs. Then, the intracavitary portion of the myoma may exfoliate elongated or fusiform groups or isolated cells of similar size with indefinite outlines and a poorly staining granular cytoplasm. Nuclei are usually absent but may be present when cellular degeneration is less advanced. Smooth muscle cells without nuclei have been called "vermiform bodies"; they are often associated with other evidence of necrosis and inflammation. Differentiation from leiomyosarcoma cells is usually not difficult.[10]

INFLAMMATIONS

The endometrium reacts to inflammatory stimuli of infectious and noninfectious nature, like any other body tissue. There is normal cyclical inflammatory response of the endometrium in the premenstrual and menstrual phases of the cycle, secondary to vascular obliteration, ischemia and necrosis of the endometrium. Endometritis related to pathologic processes is usually associated with loss of the normal cyclical characteristics of the endometrium.[21] In general, necrotic tissue, regardless of etiology, stimulates an inflammatory process. The first, or acute phase in the inflammatory process is characterized by the presence of edema, extravasated erythrocytes, polymorphonuclear leukocytes and nuclear debris. Should the inflammatory process continue on to chronicity, there will be lymphocytes, plasma cells, histiocytes and findings of a regenerative nature such as granulation tissue and fibrosis. Acute or chronic inflammatory processes are represented in smears by the presence of the aforementioned cellular elements as well as necrotic debris. Incident to such inflammatory processes, the endometrium may be disrupted and exfoliate large numbers or even sheets of epithelial cells, which can also be detected in cytologic smears. Should a granulomatous process, such as tuberculosis or a foreign body granuloma, involve the endometrium, the smear may show non-specific inflammatory cells, endometrial cells and, on rare occasion, multinucleated giant cells. The most significant problem related to granulomatous disease is the atypism of regenerating epithelial cells. In some instances, it is almost impossible by means of smear study alone to decide whether such alterations represent a regenerative or neoplastic process[6, 23] so that tissue study is an absolute necessity.

HISTIOCYTES

Another very difficult and common diagnostic problem is the smear containing an excessive number of histiocytes. Histiocytes are often encountered in conjunction with endometrial adenocarcinoma; it should be emphasized, on the other hand, that histiocytes are also pres-

ent in moderate numbers in other situations, such as immediately before and after menstruation, after delivery or abortion and in inflammatory conditions and hyperplasias. When there is a chronic inflammatory process of the endometrium, histiocytes tend to be present in large
numbers, may be slightly increased in size and often show excessive
mitotic activity. Nuclei of such histiocytic cells may be slightly hyperchromatic with an irregular chromatin pattern and usually contain 1 or
2 nucleoli. The cytoplasm is often foamy. When these cells cluster and
degenerate partially, they may be difficult to distinguish from adenocarcinoma cells. Histiocytic cells can be differentiated most readily from
cells of adenocarcinoma by careful smear analysis which traces transitional forms from normal to abnormal histiocytes.[26] The nuclear area
may also be used to differentiate histiocytes from cells of adenocarcinoma, although it is of less practical value than the just-mentioned
method. Histiocytic nuclei measure between 31.6 and 56.9 μ^2 with a
mean of 41.3 μ^2. That size is significantly smaller than cancer cell nuclei, even should the neoplasm be a well-differentiated endometrial
carcinoma. While multinucleated histiocytic cells are usually syncytial,
those of adenocarcinoma seldom show this arrangement. Other syncytial multinucleated giant cells, such as cells infected with the virus of
herpes simplex, giant endocervical cells, syncytiotrophoblast and cells
of squamous carcinoma may present diagnostic problems. Exogenous
cytoplasmic inclusions are an added factor favoring a histiocytic origin
of questionable cells.[37] It is important to understand that similar inflammatory changes can be present in either histiologic or cytologic
material[1, 16, 19, 34, 43] obtained from patients using intrauterine contraceptive devices (IUCD). There may also be epithelial atypia but this is
thought to be an unusual response to an IUCD.

Neoplastic and Non-neoplastic Conditions of the Placenta

The placenta after its initial formative stage consists of innumerable
chorionic villi that are composed of a central, vascular, mesenchymal
core covered by two layers of cells. The innermost cells form the Lang-
hans, or cytotrophoblastic, layer composed of cuboidal or polygonal
cells with centrally located nuclei; the outermost layer is called syncytiotrophoblast and is made up of multinucleated syncytial cells. Cells
covering the chorionic villi are rarely identified in routine smears from
pregnant women but may be observed in smears from patients with
placenta previa, or following abortion or delivery. The nuclei of the syncytiotrophoblast contain 10–12 heavy chromatin blocks which are irregularly dispersed within a well-defined and regular nuclear membrane. This appearance has been likened to "coarsely ground pepper."[37]

The most significant cytologic finding in patients with hydatidiform mole or choriocarcinoma is the observation of large cells with huge nuclei containing multiple, irregular, enlarged nucleoli. In addition, smears prepared from endometrial aspiration specimens in such instances may show the following[21]:

1. A very hemorrhagic background.
2. Cell syncytia that may contain up to 40 irregular, oval-shaped, small nuclei.
3. Isolated polygonal cells with large hyperchromatic nuclei.
4. Free nuclei that are large and very hyperchromatic.

RADIATION CHANGES

Uterine adenocarcinoma is considered to be sensitive to ionizing radiation, although radiation fails to eradicate carcinoma entirely in 23% of cases.[39] The observation of radiation reaction in endometrial smears is dependent to a great extent on the radiation dosage and the time following irradiation that the examination is made.

The following cellular alterations occur after weak-to-"adequate" radiation therapy. Usually at 6–8 weeks after irradiation, but in unusual circumstances as early as 2 weeks, the non-neoplastic glandular epithelial cells enlarge and develop perinuclear vacuolization, creating the appearance of a perinuclear halo. Associated with these cytologic changes, there is also evidence of acute inflammation; tumor cells show similar but more pronounced reactions with the formation of signet ring-type cells.

Cellular findings encountered with intermediate amounts of radiation are as follows: the cells are more bizarre than those observed following weak or "adequate" radiation therapy; they have enlarged or pyknotic nuclei, at times in a syncytium; leukocytes and histiocytes are present in variable numbers. With even greater amounts of radiotherapy, the endometrium undergoes complete necrosis and is replaced by a hyaline membrane, underlying which is granulation tissue containing a variable number of epithelial cells. As anticipated, smears of endometrial aspiration specimens from these patients show only histiocytes, leukocytes and red blood cells. Because cervical stenosis occurs commonly at 3 months following therapy, study by aspiration techniques may be impossible. In smears prepared from endometrial aspiration specimens, or spontaneously exfoliated material, tumor cells are usually absent even when tumor is present in the uterine wall. Thus, the success of irradiation therapy of endometrial adenocarcinoma cannot be judged adequately on the basis of cytologic findings. The cytologic changes in both uninvolved and neoplastic endometrium do not appear to differ with the type of irradiation used.[17]

REFERENCES

1. Abrams, R. Y., and Spritzer, T.: Endometrial cytology in patients using intrauterine contraceptive devices, Acta cytol. 10:240, 1966.
2. Arrighi, A. A.: Cytology of endometrial hyperplasia, Acta cytol. 2:613, 1958.
3. Atkin, N. B., Richard, B. N., and Ross, A. J.: The deoxyribonucleic acid content of carcinoma of the uterus: an assessment of its possible significance in relation to histopathology and clinical course, based on data from 165 cases, Brit. J. Cancer 13:773, 1959.
4. Boschann, H. W.: Should one routinely perform intra-uterine smears? Acta cytol. 2: 591, 1958.
5. Boschann, H. W.: The diagnostic accuracy of vaginal smears of detection of endometrial carcinoma (disc.), Acta cytol. 2:633, 1958.
6. Boschann, H. W.: Cytology of endometritis, Acta cytol. 2:524, 1958.
7. Boschann, H. W.: Cytometry on normal and abnormal endometrial cells, Acta cytol. 2: 520, 1958.
8. Boschann, H. W.: Cytology of endometrial hyperplasia (disc.), Acta cytol. 2:618, 1958.
9. deBrux, J. A., and Froment-Dupré, J.: Cytology of endometrial hyperplasia, Acta cytol. 2:613, 1958.
10. deBrux, J. A., and Froment-Dupré, J.: Cytology of endometrial polyp, Acta cytol. 2:530, 1958.
11. Evans, R. W.: *Histological Appearances of Tumors* (2d ed.; Edinburgh and London: E. & S. Livingstone, Ltd., 1966), pp. 719–48.
12. Gaudefray, M.: The diagnostic accuracy of vaginal smears for detection of endometrial carcinoma, Acta cytol. 2:582, 1958.
13. Graham, R. M.: The diagnostic accuracy of vaginal smears for detection of endometrial carcinoma, Acta cytol. 2:579, 1958.
14. Graham, R. M.: Hormonal evaluation by means of vaginal cytology of patients with endometrial carcinoma (disc.), Acta cytol. 2:631, 1958.
15. Graham, R. M.: *The Cytologic Diagnosis of Cancer* (Philadelphia: W. B. Saunders Company, 1963), p. 122.
16. Hall, H. H., Sedlis, A., Chabon, I., and Stone, M. L.: Effect of intrauterine stainless steel ring on endometrial structure and function, Am. J. Obst. & Gynec. 93:1031, 1965.
17. Haour, P., Hopman, B. C., and Terzano, G.: Advantages and disadvantages of intrauterine aspiration technique for endometrial cytology, Acta cytol. 2:566, 1958.
18. Harris, H. R.: Foam cells in the stroma of carcinoma of the body of the uterus and uterine polyp, J. Clin. Path. 11:19, 1958.
19. Havránek, F., and Králová, A.: Effect of intrauterine contraceptive device upon endometrial exfoliative cytology, lying-in, J. Reprod. Med. 1:583, 1968.
20. Hertig, A. T., and Gore, H.: *Tumors of the Female Sex Organs*, Part 2. Tumors of the Vulva, Vagina and Uterus, in *Atlas of Tumor Pathology* (Armed Forces Institute of Pathology, 1960).
21. Horava, A., DeNeef, J. C., Boutselis, J. C., and von Haam, E.: The exfoliative cytologic characteristics of the endometrium in health and disease, Obst. & Gynec. 4:1128, 1961.
22. Isaacson, P. G., Pilot, L. M. J. R., and Gooselaw, J. G.: Foam cells in the stroma in cancer of the endometrium, Obst. & Gynec. 23:9, 1964.
23. Koss, L. G.: *Diagnostic Cytology and Its Histopathologic Bases* (2d. ed.; Philadelphia and Montreal: J. B. Lippincott Company, 1968), pp. 253–56.
24. Liu, W., Barrow, M. J., Spitler, M. F., and Kochis, A. F.: Normal exfoliation of endometrial cells in pre-menopausal women, Acta cytol. 7:211, 1963.
25. Montalvo-Ruiz, L.: The diagnostic accuracy of vaginal smears for detection of endometrial carcinoma, Acta cytol. 2:582, 1958.
26. Nasiell, M.: Histiocytes and histiocytic reaction in vaginal cytology, Cancer 14:1223, 1961.
27. Ng, A. B. P.: Mixed carcinoma of the endometrium, Am. J. Obst. & Gynec. 102:506, 1968.
28. Novak, E. R., and Woodruff, J. D.: *Gynecologic and Obstetric Pathology* (5th. ed.; Philadelphia: W. B. Saunders Company, 1962), pp. 145–59.
29. Novak, E. R., and Woodruff, J. D.: *Gynecologic and Obstetric Pathology* (5th. ed.; Philadelphia: W. B. Saunders Company, 1962), pp. 202–206.

30. Nuovo, V. M.: The diagnostic accuracy of vaginal smears for detection of endometrial carcinoma, Acta cytol. 2:566, 1958.
31. Reagan, J. W., and Ng, A. B. P.: *The Cells of Uterine Adenocarcinoma* (Baltimore: Williams and Wilkins Company, 1965).
32. Roddick, J. W.: Personal communication.
33. Song, Y. S.: Cytology of endometrial polyp, Acta cytol. 2:534, 1958.
34. Tamada, T., Okagaki, T., Maruyama, M., and Matsumoto, S.: Endometrial histology associated with an intrauterine contraceptive device, Am. J. Obst. & Gynec. 98:811, 1967.
35. Tweeddale, D. N., Early, L. S., and Goodsitt, G. S.: Endometrial adenoacanthoma, Obst. & Gynec. 23:611, 1964.
36. Tweeddale, D. N., Gorthey, R. L., Harvey, H. E., and Tanner, F. H.: Cervical vs. endometrial carcinoma, Obst. & Gynec. 2:623, 1953.
37. Tweeddale, D. N., Scott, R. C., Fields, M. J., Roddick, J. W., and Ball, M. J.: Giant cells in cervico-vaginal smears, Acta cytol. 12:298, 1968.
38. von Haam, E.: The diagnostic accuracy of vaginal smears for detection of endometrial carcinoma, Acta cytol. 2:580, 1958.
39. von Haam, E.: Cytology of irradiated uterine cavity, Acta cytol. 2:546, 1958.
40. Wachtel, E.: The diagnostic accuracy of vaginal smears for detection of endometrial carcinoma, Acta cytol. 2:582, 1958.
41. Wachtel, E.: Hormonal evaluation by means of vaginal cytology of patients with endometrial carcinoma (disc.), Acta cytol. 2:630, 1958.
42. Wied, G. L.: Hormonal evaluation by means of vaginal cytology of patients with endometrial carcinoma, Acta cytol. 2:629, 1958.
43. Willson, J. R., Ledger, W. J., and Andros, G. J.: The effect of an intrauterine contraceptive device on the histologic pattern of the endometrium, Am. J. Obst. & Gynec. 93:802, 1965.

CHAPTER 16

The Cytopathology of Nonuterine Metastatic Neoplasms

Nonuterine Carcinomas

IN ORDER OF decreasing incidence, the sites of origin of metastatic neoplasms to the uterus that are demonstrable by vaginal cytology include the following: ovary (73%), fallopian tube (15%), breast (Fig. 16-1, *A* and *B*) and gastrointestinal tract (Fig. 16-1, *C*). Carcinoma of the ovary is by far the most common extrauterine neoplasm that may present in vaginal smears[8] (Fig. 16-1, *D, E* and *F*). In some cases, cells from this neoplasm are transported from the ovary via patent fallopian tubes into the uterine cavity. In other instances, the cells desquamate from metastatic tumor nodules in the uterus, fallopian tubes or vagina. Approximately one third of the women with proven ovarian carcinoma have been found to have uterine metastases at autopsy[1]; of females with clinically proven ovarian cancer, almost one third have shown ovarian tumor cells in vaginal smears.[8] In some of these cases, it is difficult to be certain whether the primary neoplasm originated in the ovary or uterus. Using cytologic material alone, it is generally not possible to indicate with certainty the primary site of metastatic neoplasm; there are, however, some cellular characteristics in smears to suggest the possibility of an ovarian tumor. For example, many ovarian tumor cells are large and contain dense nuclear chromatin that contrasts with that of most endometrial adenocarcinoma cells. Lack of the "diathesis" (necrosis, inflammation, debris and blood) in the presence of neoplastic cells should also suggest an extrauterine neoplasm (Fig. 16-1, *A*). Additionally, there is often evidence of diminished estrogen effect in smears from the lateral vaginal wall obtained from individuals with ovarian cancer. Psammoma bodies, often present in ovarian neoplasms, are occasionally observed in smear preparations[5] from such patients; on the other hand, calcific concretions may also be present in other benign or malignant neoplasms of the genital or extragenital organs.[11]

Carcinoma of the fallopian tube is a rare neoplasm and is typically a papillary adenocarcinoma. According to Sedlis,[10] a rather high percent-

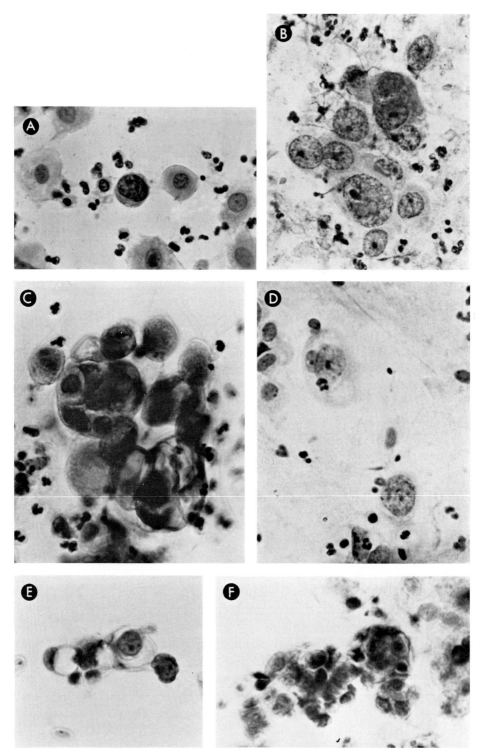

Fig. 16-1.—See legend on facing page.

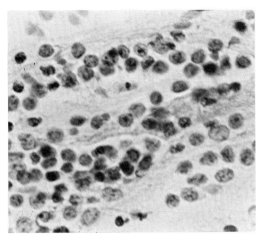

Fig. 16-2. – Cervical smear from a patient with lymphatic leukemia. The cells are fairly regular, rounded and have scant cytoplasm. Lymphocytes in cervical smears may come from lymphoid nodules of the cervix, a malignant lymphoma or leukemia.

age (40%) of women with this neoplasm will manifest positive cytologic findings. Unfortunately, cellular characteristics are not sufficiently specific to permit definite localization of fallopian tube malignancy by such means. When large adenocarcinoma cells with hyperchromatic nuclei, prominent nucleoli and cytoplasmic vacuoles are observed and no primary site is identified by cervical biopsy or endometrial curettage, carcinoma of the fallopian tube should be strongly considered.[2, 4, 9]

Other Neoplasms

Both epithelial and, less commonly, nonepithelial neoplasms originating from outside the uterus may reveal their presence in vaginal smears. Desquamated cells from Hodgkin's disease limited to the uterus have been identified, although a specific cytologic diagnosis is almost impossible.[7] Similarly, leukemic cells can be identified or suggested in vaginal smears, either with the usual cytologic stains or with the Giemsa stain (Fig. 16-2).[3, 6]

←

Fig. 16-1. – Nonuterine carcinoma. **A,** metastatic breast cancer. The single large cell in the center of the field has a large nucleus containing coarsely granular chromatin and a prominent nucleolus. This contrasts with the rest of the smear which consists mostly of parabasal cells and minimal inflammatory reaction. **B,** cervicovaginal smear from a 47-year-old woman with a widely disseminated adenocarcinoma of the breast. Obvious malignant cellular characteristics are seen. **C,** mucus-producing cells of a colonic adenocarcinoma extending into the upper vagina. In certain cases, these cells would be difficult to distinguish from those of primary endocervical adenocarcinoma. **D,** cervicovaginal smear from a woman with a large mucinous cystadenocarcinoma of the ovary. The cells at the top left have large intracytoplasmic vacuoles. The malignant cells at the bottom have altered nuclear/cytoplasmic ratios and modest clumping of nuclear chromatin. **E,** cervicovaginal smear from a 41-year-old woman with a serous cystadenocarcinoma of the ovary. Findings included positive abdominal fluid and tumor nodules in the cul-de-sac. The fairly small cells are similar to some observed from low-grade cervical, or from some endometrial adenocarcinomas. Prominent intracytoplasmic vacuoles are present. **F,** cells from the same patient as **E** which show tight groupings and an altered nuclear/cytoplasmic ratio. Squamous cells (not shown) showed some abnormalities, most likely an associated dysplasia, but biopsy proof is not available.

References

1. Abrams, H. L., Spiro, R., and Goldstein, N.: Metastasis in carcinoma. Analysis of 1,000 autopsied cases, Cancer 3:74, 1950.
2. Brewer, J. L., and Guderian, A. M.: Diagnosis of tubal cancer by vaginal cytology, Obst. & Gynec. 8:664, 1956.
3. Ceelen, G. H., and Sakurai, M.: Vaginal cytology in leukemia, Acta cytol. 6:370, 1962.
4. Fidler, H. K., and Lock, D. R.: Carcinoma of the fallopian tube detected by cervical smear, Am. J. Obst. & Gynec. 67:1103, 1954.
5. Graham, R. M., and van Niekerk, W. A.: Vaginal cytology in cancer of the ovary, Acta cytol. 6:496, 1962.
6. Luksch, F.: Leukemic cells in vaginal smears, Acta cytol. 6:95, 1962.
7. Nasiell, M.: Hodgkin's disease limited to the uterine cervix, Acta cytol. 6:16, 1962.
8. Reagan, J. W., and Ng, A. B. P.: *The Cells of Uterine Adenocarcinoma* (Baltimore: Williams and Wilkins Company, 1965).
9. Schenck, S. B., and Mackles, A.: Primary carcinoma of fallopian tubes with positive smears, Am. J. Obst. & Gynec. 81:782, 1961.
10. Sedlis, A.: Primary carcinoma of the fallopian tube, Obst. & Gynec. Surv. 16:209, 1961.
11. Tweeddale, D. N., and Pederson, B. L.: Serous neoplasms of the ovary, Am. J. M. Sc. 249:701, 1965.

CHAPTER 17

The Cytopathology of Sarcomas of the Female Genital Tract

ONLY A SMALL percentage of all malignant uterine tumors are sarcomas.[1, 10] Many classifications and subclassifications have been proposed,[8] but it is most convenient to subdivide them into the following five types: leiomyosarcomas, endometrial stromal sarcomas, mixed mesodermal tumors, sarcoma botryoides and carcinosarcomas.

Leiomyosarcoma

Leiomyosarcoma is the commonest uterine sarcoma, consisting of neoplastic smooth muscle cells of varying differentiation. Some leiomyosarcomas arise from a pre-existing leiomyoma and others arise de novo from the myometrium. Well-differentiated tumors consist of bundles or fascicles of elongated and spindle-shaped cells, resembling normal uterine smooth muscle cells. With decreasing degrees of differentiation, an increasing number of cells become round, giant in configuration and cytologically variable. Because these tumors arise within the wall of the myometrium, cells are not desquamated into the uterine cavity until the lesion is far advanced and erodes the overlying endometrium.

Our experience with the cytopathology of leiomyosarcoma is confined to one case, as follows: The initial cytologic diagnosis of a 43-year-old woman was of malignant cells, most likely squamous cell carcinoma. Her subsequent tissue diagnosis was leiomyosarcoma. A review of the original cytology slides demonstrated clustering of the neoplastic cells, at times in whorls or fascicles (Fig. 17-1). Cytoplasmic borders were indistinct between constituent cells. Most had centrally located, blunt-ended nuclei, slightly irregular in size and shape. Some isolated cells demonstrated elongated, bipolar, cyanophilic cytoplasm. The coarse and irregularly clumped nuclear chromatin varied in composition from cell to cell. Nucleoli were either very small or inapparent. Many eryth-

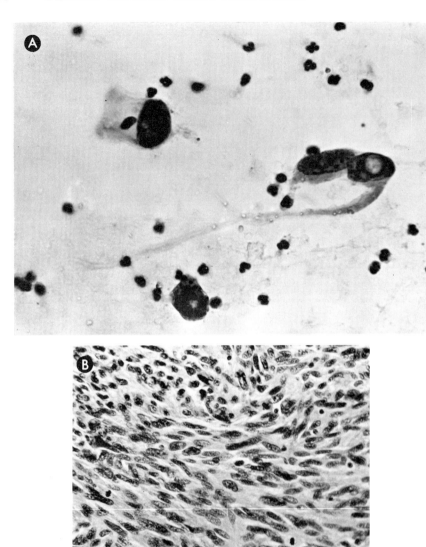

Fig. 17-1. — Leiomyosarcoma of the corpus uteri which extended into the endocervix. **A,** large cyanophilic, elongate, spindled cells have prominent nuclei with a coarsely granular chromatin pattern. There are nuclear vacuoles but no nucleoli observed. Cells with similar features are observed in some cases of keratinizing squamous cancer of the cervix. In those instances, however, there are also other neoplastic cells with more characteristic epithelial features. These cells are much larger than those encountered from uterine smooth muscle. **B,** histopathology of the patient whose cells are shown in **A.** There are numerous mitotic figures evident.

rocytes and scattered leukocytes were also noted. Histologic sections showed the leiomyosarcoma to originate in the uterine corpus with extension into the endocervical region where the overlying mucosa was eroded, thus accounting for the positive smears. On two follow-up visits, vaginal cytologic study substantiated recurrences in the vaginal cuff. The nuclear chromatin of the recurrent tumor cells was increased and denser by comparison with those from previous smear study; but such an alteration was not as evident in histologic sections. At the time of the third recurrence some months later, there were even more pleomorphic sarcoma cells in smears, many containing prominent nucleoli. There was associated hemosiderin in neoplastic cells and histiocytes. The last, and more ominous-appearing, cytosmears correlated closely with similar changes in the histologic appearance of the neoplasm.

In some cases, it is possible to suggest diagnosis of leiomyosarcoma on the basis of these desquamated cells, if the observer is thinking of this rare malady. As in the above case, it is also possible to identify a recurrence as well as a change in tumor morphology.

Endometrial Stromal Sarcoma

This neoplasm is usually a polypoid endometrial tumor composed of cells resembling those of the endometrial stroma. At times, the cells of these tumors are so undifferentiated that their stromal origin is clouded with uncertainty.[6] Neither we nor others[4] have studied smears obtained from patients with this lesion.

Mixed Mesodermal Tumor

This malignant tumor occurs usually in postmenopausal women; it is composed in a mixture of sarcomatous elements, with or without an epithelial component. The hallmark is the presence of sarcomatous elements foreign to the normal uterus, such as striated muscle cells, cartilage, osteoid or fat. Grossly, they are usually polypoid with extensive involvement of the endometrium.[2, 5] These tumors are so rare that they are seldom recognized cytologically. Thus, specific cytologic characteristics have not been adequately categorized. Most smears from mixed mesodermal sarcomas have simulated carcinoma.[5, 10] On rare occasions, an elongated cell with cytoplasmic cross-striations may be identified, to categorize with near certainty this type of neoplasm.[10] A representative case from our files was of a 38-year-old married woman who developed vaginal spotting and moderately heavy menometrorrhagia following an intrauterine pregnancy. A fungating, friable, bleeding mass so filled the vagina that it presented at the introitus. The initial cytosmear resembled endocervical adenocarcinoma (Fig. 17-2).

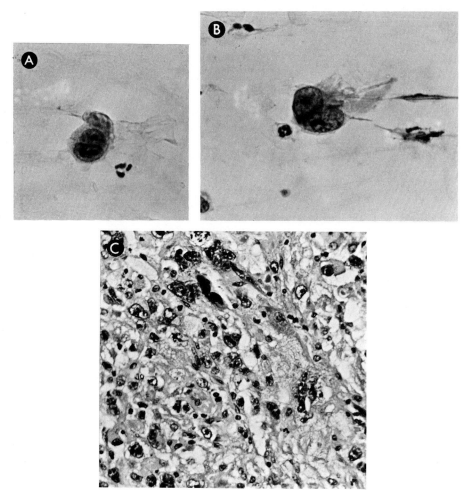

Fig. 17-2.—Mixed mesodermal tumor of the endometrial stroma. **A** and **B**, binucleated malignant cells with irregular light cyanophilic cytoplasm. Nuclear chromatin is finely granular and there are prominent nucleoli. The histopathology is shown in **C**. **C**, histologic pattern of the tumor which was composed primarily of spindled cells with considerable cytoplasm. Some cells are binucleated and many have prominent nucleoli.

Sarcoma Botryoides

Sarcoma botryoides is a variant of mixed mesodermal tumor, which is separately listed because of its unusual gross appearance and its common occurrence in infants, children or, less commonly, young women. It is characteristically polypoid, in most cases taking the form of a cluster of edematous vesicles simulating grapes.[2, 9] Because they originate in subepithelial tissues, these tumor cells seldom desquamate at an early stage of development. Neoplastic cells are variable in size and shape, although most are small, round to oval and have scant cyto-

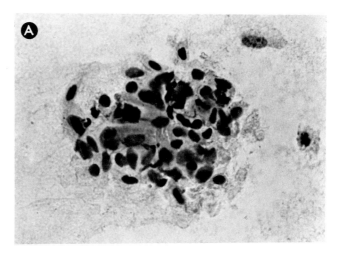

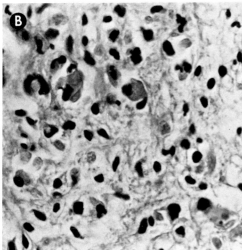

Fig. 17-3. – Sarcoma botryoides. **A,** imprint from a 32-month-old female shows a group of small, irregular cells with markedly hyperchromatic nuclei showing modest variation in size and shape. The pale cyanophilic cytoplasm does not reveal cross-striations. **B,** histologic section corresponding to the cells in **A** shows the cellular features described in **A.** Cross-striations can be seen with difficulty. The over-all picture is deceptively benign.

plasm. Some larger cells with an eccentric nucleus have cytoplasm in which striations may be identified.

Our experience with sarcoma botryoides is limited to one case in which cytologic material was available from both vaginal smears and imprints of the tumor. The 32-month-old female with a 2-month history of intermittent vaginal bleeding was found, on pelvic examination, to have grapelike masses protruding from the vaginal orifice. Vaginal smears taken after a biopsy revealed occasional small neoplastic cells. Subsequently, a total pelvic exenteration was performed. Imprints were made from the surgical specimen (Fig. 17-3). These smears demonstrated a variable number of isolated neoplastic cells, appearing deceptively benign on initial observation since they were quite small and closely resembled lymphocytes. The majority of the cells showed little variation in size. Most were round with a very narrow rim of cyanophil-ic or amphophilic cytoplasm. The nuclei were usually round and had a slightly variable, "peppery" type of chromatin pattern with a small but irregularly shaped nucleolus. Occasional cells were larger with an ec-centrically located nucleus and proportionately more cyanophilic cyto-plasm than the small cell variety. No definite intracytoplasmic stria-tions were identified in cells from cytology smears, although they were seen in tissue sections.

Carcinosarcoma of the Uterus

Uterine carcinosarcoma is a neoplasm in which there is an intimate admixture of variable amounts of carcinomatous and nonspecific sar-comatous constituents, without heterologous elements.[7] These typically polypoid, soft growths occur in postmenopausal women.

Three cases of this neoplasm were evaluated by correlating both tis-sue and cytologic material. One was in a 56-year-old postmenopausal woman with a history of continuous, slight vaginal bleeding for 3 months prior to admission. A dilatation and curettage performed else-where revealed adenocarcinoma. Shortly after admission to the Medical Center, a vaginal smear revealed adenocarcinoma cells, probably of endometrial origin (Fig. 17-4, A and B). A fractional curettage demon-strated carcinosarcoma (Fig. 17-4, C). She was treated by external ra-diation and a radical hysterectomy.

The neoplastic cells in the smears consisted of clusters of large cells with prominent cytoplasmic vacuoles. The eccentric nuclei contained increased, but finely dispersed, chromatin; nucleoli were apparent. It is understandable why only adenocarcinoma cells were seen since the tumor was predominantly an adenocarcinoma, with only small areas of sarcomatous stroma.

The second carcinosarcoma was a necrotic tumor composed predomi-nantly of pleomorphic sarcomatous elements associated with only scat-tered neoplastic glands (Fig. 17-5, A and B). The smear showed much necrosis, inflammation and many pleomorphic neoplastic cells. The majority of these cells were isolated, although some were clustered into small groups. The generally single and slightly eccentric nuclei were of variable chromatin content and contained prominent, single or double nucleoli (Fig. 17-5, C and D).

The third case was a 60-year-old single woman who had had "radium treatment" for excessive vaginal bleeding at age 38. That treatment led to the development of menopausal symptoms and amenorrhea. Five months prior to her most recent admission, she developed profuse wa-tery, pink, occasionally blood-stained vaginal discharge and complained of lower abdominal discomfort. Admission examination revealed an enlarged, soft uterus.

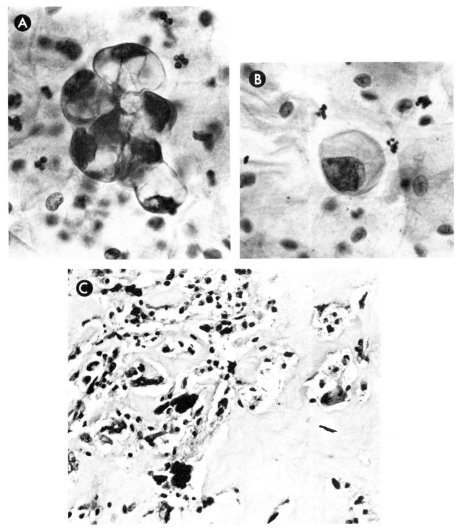

Fig. 17-4. – Carcinosarcoma of the endometrial stroma in a 56-year-old postmenopausal female. **A**, a group of cells most likely from the glandular part of the neoplasm. **B**, a single large neoplastic cell probably from the sarcomatous area. **C**, histologic section from the sarcomatous area. There are both single and grouped cells in the collagenous stroma, some are spindled, whereas others are rounded.

The vaginal smears were very bloody and contained many neoplastic cells in loose, large clusters as well as some that were isolated. The malignant elements were generally large cells with the nucleus occupying a large proportion of total cell area. Nuclei were oval to round, often irregular and contained a slightly coarse chromatin pattern and prominent nucleoli. A pale blue cytoplasm had indistinct borders, especially in clustered cells. In essence, cellular elements were those of undifferentiated malignant cells. The excised uterus was enlarged, markedly

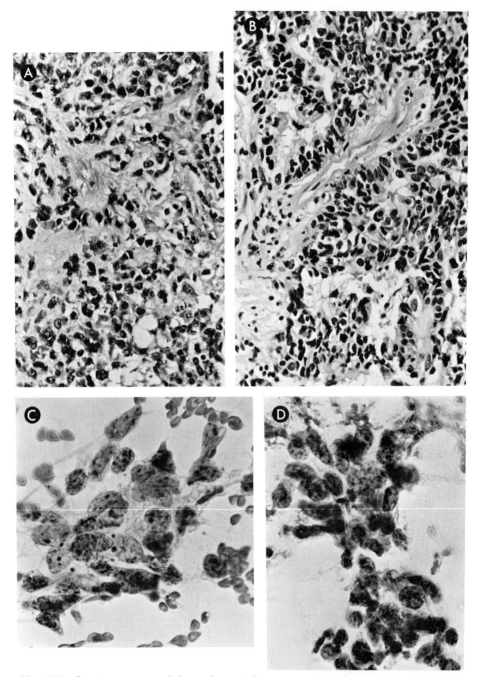

Fig. 17-5. — Carcinosarcoma of the endometrial stroma. **A,** histologic section from a sarcomatous area. The cells are slightly variable in size and irregular or spindled, corresponding to those seen in **B. B,** histologic section from a carcinomatous area showing irregular gland formation. The smear cells shown in **D** relate to this histologic pattern. **C,** most cells encountered in this lesion are larger than those seen in endometrial adenocarcinoma. Some seen in this smear have fairly long cytoplasmic processes and resemble the cells of sarcoma. **D,** clusters of malignant cells similar to some encountered in adenocarcinoma. These cells probably came from the malignant glandular portion of the tumor shown in **B.**

distorted and showed complete replacement of the endometrium by a pink-tan necrotic neoplasm extending deeply into the myometrium. Histologic examination of the tumor revealed a variegated pattern in which very cellular sarcomatous elements predominated plus a lesser component of scattered foci of glandular neoplastic structures and malignant squamous epithelium.

Our experience indicates that it is possible to identify lesions as sarcomas by cytology but, because of the paucity with which we see them, it is seldom possible to identify the specific variety by cytologic means. Cytology may be valuable in detecting recurrent sarcomas.

REFERENCES

1. Bautselis, J. G., and Ullery, J. C.: Sarcoma of the uterus, Obst. & Gynec. 20:28, 1962.
2. Evans, R. W.: *Histological Appearances of Tumors* (2d ed.; Edinburgh and London: E. & S. Livingstone, Ltd., 1966), pp. 57–62.
3. Holmquest, N. D.: The exfoliative cytology of mixed mesodermal tumors of the uterus, Acta cytol. 6:373, 1962.
4. Koss, L. G.: *Diagnostic Cytology and Its Histopathologic Bases* (2d ed.; Philadelphia and Montreal: J. B. Lippincott Company, 1968), pp. 262–64.
5. Norris, H. J., Roth, E., and Taylor, H. B.: Mesenchymal tumors of the uterus. II. A clinical and pathologic study of 31 mixed mesodermal tumors, Obst. & Gynec. 28:57, 1966.
6. Norris, H. J., and Taylor, H. B.: Mesenchymal tumors of the uterus. I. A clinical and pathological study of 53 endometrial stromal tumors, Cancer 19:755, 1966.
7. Norris, H. J., and Taylor, H. B.: Mesenchymal tumors of the uterus. III. A clincial and pathologic study of 31 carcinosarcomas, Cancer 19:1459, 1966.
8. Ober, W. B.: Uterine sarcomas: histogenesis and taxonomy, Ann. New York Acad. Sc. 75:568, 1959.
9. Ober, W. B., and Edgcomb, J. H.: Sarcoma Botryoides in the female urogenital tract, Cancer 7:75, 1954.
10. Parker, J. E.: Cytologic findings associated with primary uterine malignancies of mixed cell types (malignant mixed müllerian tumor), Acta cytol. 8:316, 1964.

CHAPTER 18

The Cytopathology of Primary
Vaginal and Vulvar Neoplasms

Primary Vaginal Neoplasms

Vaginal tumors represent 1% to 2% of all cancers of the female genital tract.[5, 7] Most (70%) are invasive squamous cell cancers and the majority of the remainder are carcinomas in situ.[5] Slightly over 50% of the in situ neoplasms will be exclusively vaginal; that is, they do not accompany or follow a similar lesion of the cervix. Other primary malignancies of the vagina are exceedingly rare and include malignant melanoma, adenocarcinoma and botyroid sarcomas.

Primary In Situ Squamous Cell Carcinoma
of the Vagina

Most primary vaginal in situ cancers are located in the upper portion of that organ.[5] Such lesions may occasionally be observed in the middle or lower vagina or may be multicentric. Should cytologic study be positive in the absence of a visible lesion and should the cervix show no malignancy on biopsy, it would be wise to investigate the possibility of in situ cancer of the vagina.

Cytologic findings indicative of carcinoma in situ of the vagina are identical with those for in situ cancer of other sites, i.e., the cervix. The precise location of vaginal lesions may be difficult to delineate, necessitating use of fractionated cytologic specimens (from upper, middle and lower vagina, separately labeled), or staining with Schiller's iodine or toluidine blue.

Invasive Squamous Cell Carcinoma of the Vagina

In most instances, invasive squamous cell cancer in the vagina represents an extension from a primary lesion of the cervix. The rare primary invasive squamous cell cancer of the vagina is usually located in the upper third; the neoplasm is ulcerative or nodular.[5, 7] Multicentricity may occur in almost 17% of such cases.[4]

Cytologic smears contain cells resembling those seen in invasive squamous cancer from other sites, such as the cervix. Because these vaginal cancers are of lower grades of malignancy, they will generally be better differentiated than those of cervical origin. However, neither cytologic or histologic features can be relied upon to delineate the origin of a neoplasm. Instead, carefully selected biopsies from identified sites should act as referee.

Miscellaneous Primary Vaginal Malignancies

Primary malignant melanoma of the vagina is a rare neoplasm.[3] Cytologic study will not be diagnostic until the tumor mass has caused ulceration of the vaginal mucosa. By then it is usually symptomatic and has often extended beyond the limits of resectability. The cells of malignant melanoma are variable in size; their shapes are elliptical to irregular. Cytoplasm is pale blue and may or may not contain small, variously sized melanin granules. Nuclei, occupying at least 50% of mean cell area, are often eccentrically situated. Nuclear chromatin is generally coarse; one to two prominent nucleoli are common (Fig. 18-1).

Fig. 18-1. – Myriads of malignant melanoma cells of different sizes. The largest cell contains innumerable melanin granules of varying size. Other cells have clear-to-light cyanophilic cytoplasm without the presence of melanin granules. The nuclear/cytoplasmic ratio is large. Finely granular nuclei almost always contain one or two recognizable nucleoli.

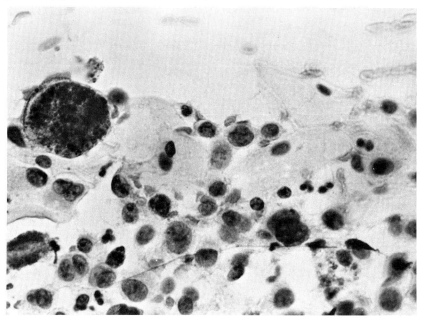

Sarcomas are either of mixed mesodermal nature, presenting as polypoid, grape-like masses in infants and rarely in adults, or are of a single mesodermal structure indigenous to the vagina, i. e., smooth muscle, fibrous tissue or blood vessels. The aforementioned will usually be large and symptomatic, before overlying vaginal mucosa ulcerates, so that cytodiagnosis assumes a purely secondary role. Smears from sarcoma botyroides show undifferentiated, irregular malignant cells with pale blue cytoplasm. Cross-striations in the cytoplasm are exceedingly difficult to identify. Nuclear findings are classic for malignancy; nucleoli are rarely encountered (see Chapt. 17).

ASSOCIATION OF VAGINAL CARCINOMA (IN SITU OR INVASIVE) WITH OTHER NEOPLASMS OF THE FEMALE GENITAL TRACT

The association between cervical and vaginal neoplasia has been previously discussed. Squamous cancers of the vulva and vagina are even more commonly combined. For example Moertel and associates[6] demonstrated that of 137 patients with cancer of the vulva or vagina, 5.8% had two or more discrete lesions of those organs. Similarly, Abell and Gosling[1] noted that 4.2% of patients with carcinoma in situ of the vulva had associated squamous vaginal cancer. One of our patients had a positive vaginal cytology 8 years after vulvectomy for invasive squamous cancer of the vulva. Investigation to determine the source of a positive cytologic smear revealed an intraepithelial cancer of the lower vagina extending into the Bartholin's duct; eventual involvement of a hemorrhoid by the same process was discovered. Cytologic findings from the aforementioned are like similar lesions of the cervix.

Primary Vulvar Neoplasms

Cancer of the vulva is an uncommon neoplasm. For example, ovarian cancer, accounting for 15% to 17% of all gynecologic malignancies, is five times more common than vulvar cancer.[8] Vulvar malignancies are usually invasive squamous cancers, commonly accompanied by in situ cancer. In situ cancer may, at times, be present as the only lesion. Invasive cancers are clinically evident so that cytology should not be relied on for diagnosis. Negative cytologic smears from ulcerative vulvar lesions do not exclude cancer.[2] Carcinoma in situ of the vulva, commonly associated with leukoplakia, ordinarily shows visible changes of the epithelium. Again, cytology assumes a secondary role to tissue biopsy. The above vulvar lesions have cytologic changes similar to squamous cancer arising in other sites.

At times, rare vulvar lesions such as adenocarcinoma, adenoacanthoma, melanoma or sarcoma, may occur. In those instances, cytologic study is only of didactic value.

REFERENCES

1. Abell, M. R., and Gosling, J. R. G.: Intraepithelial and infiltrative carcinoma of the vulva: Bowen's type, Cancer 14:318, 1961.
2. Carter, B., Kaufmann, L. A., and Cuyler, W. K.: Smear preparations in the diagnosis of vulvar carcinoma, Surg. Gynec. & Obst. 91:600, 1950.
3. Ehrmann, R. L., Younge, P. A., and Lerch, V. L.: The exfoliative cytology and histogenesis of an early malignant melanoma of the vagina, Acta cytol. 6:245, 1962.
4. Livingstone, R. G.: *Primary Carcinoma of the Vagina* (Springfield, Ill.: Charles C Thomas, Publisher, 1950).
5. Merrill, J. A., and Bender, W. T.: Primary carcinoma of the vagina, Obst. & Gynec. 11:3, 1958.
6. Moertel, C. G., Dockerty, M. B., and Baggenstoss, A. H.: Multiple primary malignant neoplasms, Cancer 14:221, 1961.
7. Rutledge, F.: Cancer of the vagina, Am. J. Obst. & Gynec. 97:635, 1967.
8. Tweeddale, D. N., and Pederson, B. L.: Serous neoplasms of the ovary (with observations on related neoplasms), Am. J. M. Sc. 249:701, 1965.

CHAPTER 19

The Cytopathology of Recurrent Carcinoma

WE WILL INCLUDE in this chapter observations on multicentric squamous neoplasia in combination with squamous cancer (in situ or invasive) of the cervix.

Careful observation after therapy for malignancy is a necessity if recurrent disease is to be recognized and eradicated. A clinically obvious recurrence offers no problem in diagnosis. However, to identify recurrent lesions as early as possible, especially since one fourth to one third may be localized,[7, 10] use of cytologic study at follow-up examinations may be invaluable. Recurrences following radiation therapy for invasive cervical carcinoma may not only mirror the original lesion, but also may reappear in the in situ stage. Whether the in situ cancer is a new cancer, a recurrence or a multicentric focus is conjectural. In addition, while an in situ cervical carcinoma is usually cured by hysterectomy, it, too, may recur or persist in the vagina following surgery.[15] Any or all of the above-noted lesions may appear months or years after initial therapy. Therefore, it is mandatory to follow such patients at regular intervals, using all practical means of observation. Since recurrent, invasive cervical carcinoma may be cytologically negative, a negative Papanicolaou smear should not impart a false sense of security. A smear is never a substitute for careful clinical examination.

Cytopathology of Recurrent Squamous Cancer Following Radiation Therapy

RADIATION CHANGES

It is necessary that the cytologist be familiar with changes induced in normal squamous or columnar epithelium by ionizing rays, since interpretation of radiation or postradiation smears is difficult. In the first few weeks of radiation therapy for cervical carcinoma, the following cellular changes occur in normal squamous (or columnar) epithelium[9, 12]:

1. Marked cellular enlargement, particularly of basal and parabasal cells, accompanied by a proportionate nuclear enlargement (Fig. 19-1, *A* and *B*).
2. A peculiar "wrinkling" of the nuclei and chromatin clumping (Fig. 19-1, *A* and *B*).
3. Vacuolization of the cytoplasm or, occasionally, of the nucleus (Fig. 19-1, *A* and *C*).
4. Multinucleation (Fig. 19-1, *A* and *B*).
5. Bizarre shapes, particularly of nuclei (Fig. 19-1, *B*).
6. Cytoplasmic acidophilia or polychromasia.

These changes may be a guide to prognosis.[9] For example, some reports[9] indicate that after therapy, if over 70% of superficial cells show this key radiation effect (RR), the response is regarded as prognostically favorable. Unfortunately, these results are hard to duplicate; for that reason, we do not routinely assess RR in our laboratory. Knowledge that such "immediate" radiation effect may occasionally persist up to 35 years[9, 11] may avoid diagnostic error (particularly overcall) of smears taken some time after completion of treatment.

Cancer cells often show marked degenerative changes during therapy and usually disappear by 3 weeks (Fig. 19-2).[22] Persistence of malignant cells for several weeks after completion of treatment, with rare exceptions, portends an ominous prognosis.[12] In unusual instances, such patients may fail to show recurrence for years.[24] As a general rule, posttreatment patients with benign cellular findings, in smears with a fairly clean background, have a better prognosis than those with nonmalignant cellular abnormalities (such as the presence of inflammatory cells, parabasal cell changes, parabasal cell changes with inflammation, dysplasia with inflammation, denuded nuclei and spindle cells or other atypical cells and inflammation). Obviously, the outlook for patients with frankly malignant cells in smears is worse than for those with nonmalignant cellular abnormalities. The identification and biologic capability of malignant cells is unquestionably difficult in many cases. For example, malignant cells may show varying degrees of radiation effect, associated with viability that is ambiguous. Additionally, posttreatment smears with malignant cells, as well as with nonmalignant cellular abnormalities, show a very high percentage of inflammatory elements. The presence of inflammatory cells may cause cellular alterations which compound an already difficult cytodiagnosis, as well as be so prevalent as to dilute the number of diagnostic cells.

Certain changes may be anticipated in the maturation index following radiation therapy. Postmenopausal women ordinarily show only minor changes in the maturation pattern. Such treatment to the cervix of premenopausal women, however, causes profound cellular changes and usually leads to a pattern similar to that of normal postmenopausal

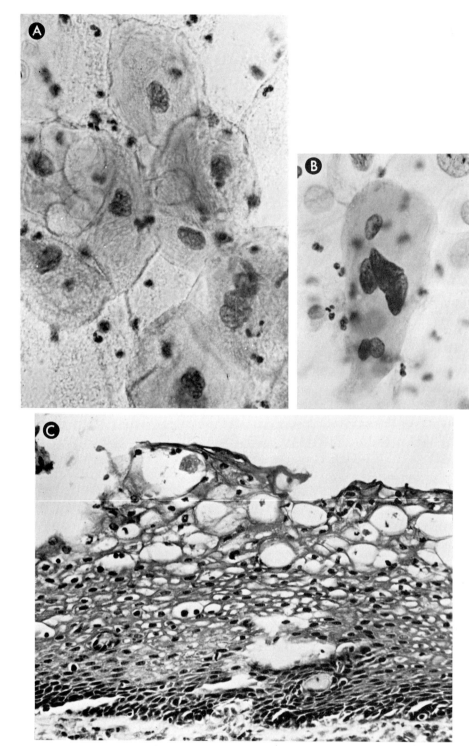

Fig. 19-1. — See legend on facing page.

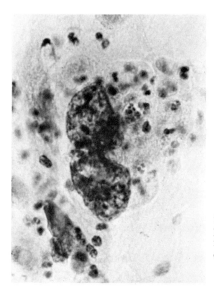

Fig. 19-2. – A cell from a smear taken in the immediate postradiotherapy period. This is most likely a radiated squamous cancer cell.

women (Fig. 19-3). Eosinophilia and nuclear pyknosis, with the appearance of superficial squamous cells, occur especially in the first months after therapy. This is followed by a gradual increase in cells of intermediate type. In the 3rd month, a parabasal pattern appears, similar to that seen after the menopause.[21] Such a parabasal picture has been regarded due to factors other than simple ovarian ablation by radiation, since it has been contended that those cells may not be responsive to estrogen.[17] Recent experience dictates that in both young and old women a parabasal pattern may be stimulated to a mature appearance by exogenous estrogen, generally in proportion to the time lapse following radiotherapy. Similarly, a right shift* in the maturation pattern may occur in younger women who are not the recipients of exogenous hormone therapy. Retention of an estrogenic cytologic pattern has been regarded as a poor prognostic sign,[23] but this is not proven. Additionally, the common association of inflammatory cells in posttreatment cytologic preparations makes assessment of a maturation index less than optimal.

*Maturation index based on percentage of *parabasal/intermediate/superficial* cells. A left shift indicated more basal cells; a right shift indicates more superficial cells.

←

Fig. 19-1. – Cellular changes following radiation therapy for cervical carcinoma. **A,** squamous cells showing characteristic radiation reactions (RR). The patient received previous radiation therapy for one month. Note the large size of the cells, the multinucleation and the prominent vacuoles. **B,** a large, benign multinucleated squamous cell following radiation therapy. Despite the ominous appearance, the large nuclear/cytoplasmic ratio is inconsistent with malignancy. **C,** histologic section of radiated squamous epithelium. Note the prominent intraepithelial vacuoles.

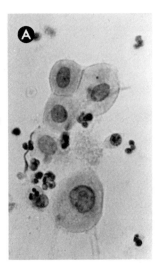

Fig. 19-3. – Cellular changes following radiation therapy. **A,** this parabasal pattern is a common sequel of radiotherapy. It usually appears in the third month, but may change so that superficial cells eventually predominate. **B,** flattened squamous epithelium commonly seen following radiotherapy. The constituent cells are often seen in large sheets in cytologic smears. The large cells contain prominent nucleoli (see Fig. 19-9*A*).

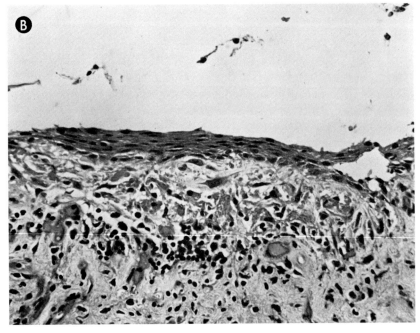

→

Fig. 19-4. – Postirradiation dysplasia. **A,** a group of large cells from a 48-year-old woman who had radiotherapy for stage I squamous cancer of the cervix 3 months previously. Two years later, she still had dysplastic cells in cervicovaginal smears. **B** and **C,** vaginal biopsy from the patient whose cells are shown in **A.** The postirradiation dysplastic reaction is mild. Polypoid vaginal dysplasia, which is not uncommon, is seen in **B. D** and **E,** small postirradiation dysplastic cells from a 69-year-old woman who was irradiated for squamous cancer of the cervix 2 years previously. Contrast the small size of these cells with those in **A. F,** biopsy from the patient whose cells are shown in **D** and **E.** The dysplastic reaction is composed of cells which are generally smaller than those seen in **B** and **C.**

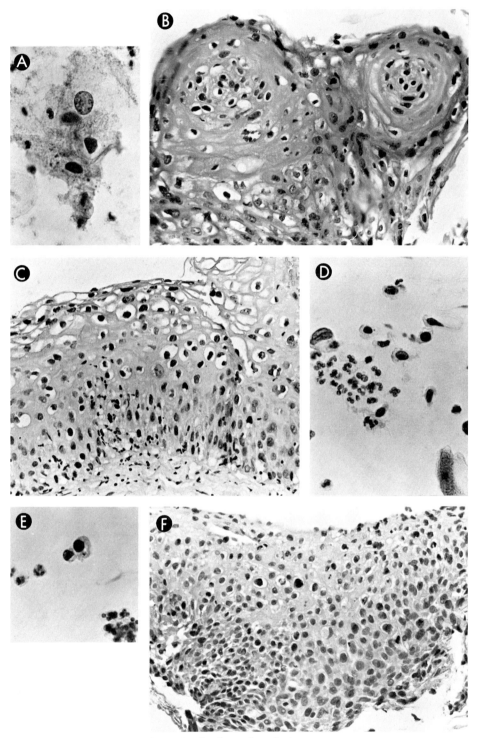

Fig. 19-4. — See legend on facing page.

Postirradiation Dysplasia of the Uterine Cervix and Vagina

Following radiotherapy for cervical neoplasia, the cervicovaginal mucosa usually displays the predictable secondary cellular alterations previously detailed. However, in almost one-third of the cases, either the cervical or vaginal mucosa may develop a dysplastic lesion. Sporadic cases have been reported in which the dysplasia has followed treatment of in situ squamous cell cancer by radiation, but it is rarely encountered after surgical therapy. It has been shown that the appearance of dysplasia in the first 2 years after therapy is associated with a significantly greater probability that cancer will recur.[19]

Cells from postirradiation dysplasia are intermediate in size between those of classic dysplasia and those of carcinoma in situ. Similarly, mean nuclear areas and nuclear cellular areas occupy the same intermediate size. In general, two major cell patterns present, a large and a small cell variety (Fig. 19-4). The various sizes are probably related to presence or absence of ovarian function, since older people have smaller cells, and the smaller cell size is related inversely to the maturation index. Individual cells are either nonisodiametric or isodiametric, the former being somewhat more frequent than the usual isodiametric cell pattern of classic dysplasia. Postirradiation dysplastic cells are about equally divided into those appearing singly or in groupings (compare Fig. 19-4, *A* and *E*) but not as syncytial masses, while cells of ordinary dysplasia are almost always isolated. A finely granular nuclear pattern is common to cells of typical and of postirradiation dysplasia. However, while the cytoplasm of the former is overwhelmingly basophilic, in the latter instance it is predominantly eosinophilic or indeterminate.

Histologic sections from postirradiation dysplasia show surface reactions similar to those from nonradiated persons. At times, despite judicious use of Schiller's iodine, it may be difficult to identify the precise vaginal location of the epithelial abnormality. Some reported cases resemble in situ cancer more than dysplasia.[18]

Postirradiation Carcinoma In Situ of the Cervix or Vagina

It is problematical whether a sharp distinction can be made between certain cases of severe postirradiation dysplasia and carcinoma in situ of the cervix or vagina. For example, Patten and co-workers[18] suggested that the 7 cases of in situ cancer of the vagina, reported by Koss and associates[13] following radiotherapy for invasive cancer closely resemble postirradiation dysplasia. However, Patten's figures 10 and 11[18] could conceivably be interpreted as in situ cancer. Bret and Coupez[3] reported one case of a microinvasive cervical cancer, treated by radical surgery and radiation, that was almost immediately followed by the appearance of positive cytologic changes. In situ cancer was verified histologically from the upper vagina. Rutledge[20] reported his experience with 25 cases of postirradiation lesions of the vagina resembling in situ cancers. In 10 of his 25 patients with 3-year follow-ups only 1 died of cancer. This benign course differs significantly from the more ominous one that follows postirradiation dysplasia. The in situ cervical or vaginal carcinomas following radiation for invasive cervical squamous cancer may originate from persistent carcinoma in situ, enhanced predisposition of remaining vaginal mucosa or incitation by irradiation.[5]

Cytologic findings in patients with postirradiation carcinoma in situ of the cervix or vagina usually resemble those of classic in situ cancer. The cells will usually be isodiametric and resemble parabasal cells. However, other cell types, particularly keratinizing cells, may be found as a result of the dry, atrophic vaginal milieu.

Histologic findings are those classic for in situ cancer. In certain instances, the site of the tissue abnormality may defy identification.

Fig. 19-5.—Recurrent cancer. **A,** pretreatment smear of an invasive large-cell, nonkeratinizing type of cervical squamous cancer. **B,** smear from the same patient as **A** taken six months later and indicating a recurrence. Note the similarity of the cell types. **C,** pretreatment smear of an invasive keratinizing squamous cell cancer of the cervix. **D,** smear from the same patient as **C** taken 9 months later and evidencing recurrent keratinizing cancer. Cell types are similar.

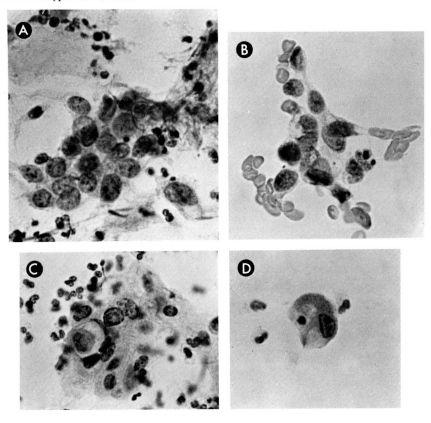

Recurrent Postirradiation Invasive Squamous Cancer of the Cervix

As stated previously, cytology is an invaluable partner with clinical examination in follow-up of previously treated cervical cancers. Absolute familiarity with radiation changes is indispensable in order to avoid an erroneous cytodiagnosis of malignancy. Routine posttreatment cytologic studies may initially establish the diagnosis of early invasive lesions. In most circumstances, however, a recurrence is clinically obvious so that cytologic studies are merely of didactic value.

Analysis of the cells of recurrent cancer usually reveals close mimicry of neoplastic elements observed in initial pretreatment smears; cancers originally of either large, nonkeratinizing or keratinizing varieties recur as the original cell type (Fig. 19-5). On occasion, the recurrence of an initially cytodiagnosed nonkeratinizing cancer may show keratinizing cancer cells, or vice versa. Such findings may merely reflect cell type variability in different areas of the tumor, although it is possible that a different cell clone gained ascendancy, possibly due to the influence of ionizing rays. As in primary cervical cancer, cells from recurrent neoplasia may be difficult to identify due to associated blood or debris. Should necrotic debris be present without tumor cells, a careful clinical search may reveal recurrent neoplasm.

Multicentric Involvement by Malignancy in Other Sites of the Female Genital Tract Following Radiotherapy for Squamous Cancer of the Cervix

About 1.1% of patients with cervical cancer will also have a squamous cell cancer of the vulva or vagina.[16] This association supports the field theory of cancer origin. Our experience with combined cervical and vulvar cancer is limited to 2 cases. In 1 patient, the lesions were synchronous; the cervical cancer was invasive while that of the vulva was in situ. Subsequent involvement of a hemorrhoid with in situ cancer occurred (Fig. 19-6). The other case was asynchronous, with invasive cancers occurring 19 years apart, the cervical lesion antedating that of the vulva.

Cytologic features of vulvar neoplasia are delineated in another section.

Only a few cases of synchronous or asynchronous invasive cancer of the cervix and vagina have been reported. It is exasperatingly difficult to document that the vaginal lesion is not either a metastasis or a recurrence of the cervical cancer. The cellular picture reveals malignant squamous elements with variable differentiation. In general, vaginal cancer is characterized by cells with less anaplasia than those originating from primary cervical squamous malignancy.

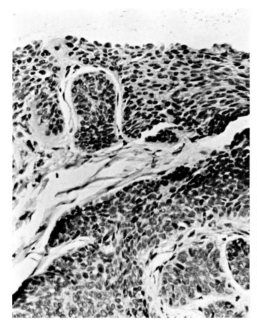

Fig. 19-6.—Microinvasive squamous cancer in a hemorrhoid from a 55-year-old woman. Nine years previously, she had a vulvectomy for squamous cancer of the vulva. In addition to the subsequent cancer involving the hemorrhoidal area, in situ cancer was also found in the lower vagina, even involving Bartholin's duct.

Cytopathology of Vaginal Squamous Cancer Following Surgical Therapy for Carcinoma In Situ of the Cervix

It is axiomatic that routine vaginal cytologic studies *should not* be discontinued following optimal surgical treatment for carcinoma in situ of the cervix. These patients must be followed by smears at least once a year for the rest of their lives. Either in situ or early invasive cancer of the vagina may be discovered by such means.

SUBSEQUENT IN SITU CANCER OF THE VAGINA

Carcinoma in situ of the vagina following hysterectomy for carcinoma in situ of the cervix is detected by cytologic study in 1%–2% of such patients.[6, 14] The vaginal lesion may be an extension, or a "seeding," of the vaginal mucosa from the cervical one, a coexistent multicentric neoplastic focus or represent a new cancer developing in a fertile environment. Slightly less than one-half of all cases of in situ cancer of the vagina appear following hysterectomy for carcinoma in situ of the cervix. Reports of such occurrences are usually limited to isolated studies,[2, 3, 6, 8, 15] although Rutledge[20] collected 14 such cases. The following composite analysis of reported cases includes 2 of our own. In 19 (73%) of 26 cases, the lesions were asynchronous with the vaginal lesion appearing 1 to 10 years after surgical therapy for the cervical neoplasm. The other 7 patients (27%) had cancers that were essentially synchronous, with both the cervical and vaginal in situ cancers being

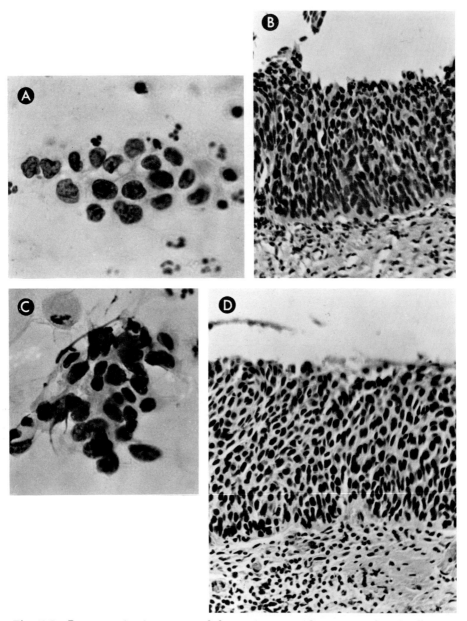

Fig. 19-7.—Recurrent in situ cancer of the vagina. **A**, malignant parabasal cells representing cancer in situ of the cervix. **B**, histologic section corresponding to the cells in **A**. This patient had a synchronous in situ cancer of the cervix as shown in **C** and **D**. **C**, malignant squamous epithelial cells in a vaginal smear taken seven weeks after a total hysterectomy for the in situ cancer of the cervix. **D**, section from the vaginal biopsy which shows carcinoma in situ. There were six such multicentric areas in the entire vaginectomy specimen.

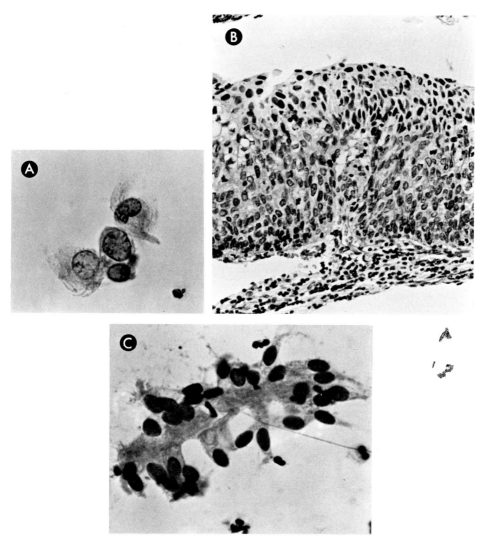

Fig. 19-8. — Recurrent in situ cancer of the vagina in a 60-year-old woman who had a hysterectomy for in situ cancer of the cervix. **A**, malignant cells which appeared in a vaginal smear a few months following the diagnosis and treatment of the cervix carcinoma. **B**, histologic section of one of the multiple areas of vaginal in situ cancer. **C**, columnar, mucus-producing cells for a vaginal smear of the same patient in **A** and **B** following a vaginectomy and colonic vaginal graft. The colonic mucosal cells closely resemble those normally encountered in the endocervix. The vaginectomy was performed for multicentric in situ cancer synchronous with cervical squamous in situ cancer. Two years later a tumor nodule of squamous cancer was noted in the vaginal apex, apparently secondary to implantation of tumor cells at the time of vaginectomy.

diagnosed within a year's time. Most (19 or 73%) were located in the vaginal apex, with 2 in the lower vagina; one was multicentric, another in the mid vagina and one extended the entire length of the vagina; in 2, the location was not stated. Radiation, partial or complete vaginectomy were the modalities of treatment. Only 12 patients were followed as long as 3 years after diagnosis; only one showed signs of further neoplasia (see Fig. 19-8).

Few details of cytologic studies of these cases are recorded. Our experience dictates that cells of in situ cancer of the vagina following hysterectomy for carcinoma in situ of the cervix generally resemble those of the cervical lesion (isodiametric, parabasal-like cells) (Figs. 19-7 and 19-8). Fractionated cytologic specimens from upper, middle or lower vagina may greatly facilitate in locating the lesion.

Histologic study reveals the classic findings of carcinoma in situ of the cervix. The use of Schiller's iodine or toluidine blue staining may assist in localizing the epithelial abnormality for optimal management.

Invasive Cancer of the Vagina Following Surgical Treatment for In Situ Cancer of the Cervix

There are only scattered reports of invasive squamous cancer of the vagina following treatment of intraepithelial cervical carcinoma.[4, 6, 8] Vaginal lesions of this type have been observed in 0.73% to 0.85% of patients with carcinoma in situ of the cervix and have appeared in the vagina from 5 months to 7½ years after treatment of the cervical neoplasm. In 2 of the 3 reported cases, follow-up was recorded, with an unfavorable outcome.[4, 6, 8] It must be added that verification of these second primary vaginal cancers depends on a careful analysis of the cervical in situ epithelioma. One must be assured that the latter lesion is not focally invasive and in continuity with the vaginal cancer.

Cytologic findings of invasive squamous cancer of the vagina are discussed in Chapter 18.

In Situ Cervical Cancer Associated with Multicentric Involvement by Malignancy in Other Sites

There is no significant association between in situ cervical cancer and other neoplasms of the female genital tract, except for the vaginal lesions previously discussed. In areas other than the female genital tract, a unique combination with cancer of the ororespiratory tract exists.[1] One and a half per cent of patients with in situ or invasive cervical cancer have shown ororespiratory tract cancer. However, almost one-fifth of females with ororespiratory cancer have cervical malignancy. All cancers were squamous (Fig. 19-9). This relationship probably

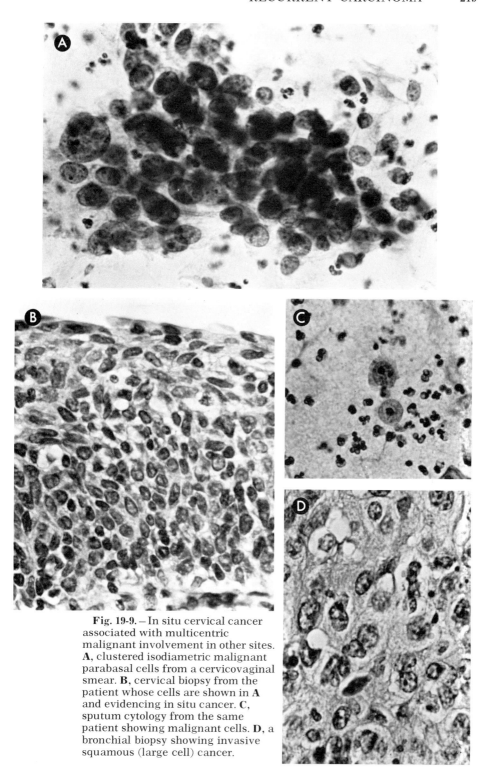

Fig. 19-9. — In situ cervical cancer associated with multicentric malignant involvement in other sites. **A**, clustered isodiametric malignant parabasal cells from a cervicovaginal smear. **B**, cervical biopsy from the patient whose cells are shown in **A** and evidencing in situ cancer. **C**, sputum cytology from the same patient showing malignant cells. **D**, a bronchial biopsy showing invasive squamous (large cell) cancer.

reflects a combination of early onset of coitus and smoking, primarily among patients from a low socioeconomic level.

References

1. Barron, S. L., Roddick, J. W., Jr., Greenlaw, R. H., Rush, B., and Tweeddale, D. N.: Multiple primary cancers of the oro-respiratory tract and the cervix, Cancer 21:672, 1968.
2. Blumberg, J. M., and Ober, W. B.: Carcinoma in situ of the cervix: recurrence in the vaginal vault. Report of a case, Am. J. Obst. & Gynec. 66:421, 1953.
3. Bret, A. J., and Coupez, J. F.: Four cases of vaginal recurrences of invasive or intraepithelial carcinoma of the uterine cervix, Acta cytol. 7:277, 1963.
4. Carter, B., Cuyler, W. K., Kaufmann, L. A., Thomas, W. L., Creadick, R. N., Parker, R. T., Peete, C. H., Jr., and Cherny, W. B.: Clinical problems in stage 0 (intraepithelial) cancer of the cervix, Am. J. Obst. & Gynec. 71:634, 1956.
5. Copenhaver, E. H., Salzman, F. A., and Wright, K. A.: Carcinoma in situ of the vagina, Am. J. Obst. & Gynec. 89:962, 1964.
6. Fennell, R. H., Jr.: Carcinoma in situ of the uterine cervix, Cancer 9:374, 1956.
7. Graham, J. B., and Meigs, J. V.: Earlier detection of recurrent cancer of the uterine cervix by vaginal smear, Am. J. Obst. & Gynec. 64:908, 1952.
8. Graham, J. B., and, Meigs, J. V.: Recurrence of tumor after total hysterectomy for carcinoma in situ, Am. J. Obst. & Gynec. 64:1159, 1952.
9. Graham, R. M.: *The Cytologic Diagnosis of Cancer* (Philadelphia and London: W. B. Saunders Company, 1963).
10. Graham, R. M.: Cytology in the treated cancer patient, Acta cytol. 8:3, 1964.
11. Kaufman, R. R., Topek, N. H., and Wall, J. A.: Late irradiation changes in vaginal cytology, Am. J. Obst. & Gynec. 81:859, 1961.
12. Koss, L. G.: *Diagnostic Cytology and Its Histopathologic Bases* (2d ed.; Philadelphia and Montreal: J. B. Lippincott Company, 1968).
13. Koss, L. G., Melamed, M. L., and Daniel, W. W.: In situ epidermoid cancer of cervix and vagina following radiotherapy for cervical cancer, Cancer 14:353, 1961.
14. Krieger, J. S., and McCormack, L. J.: Graded treatment for in situ carcinoma of the uterine cervix, Am. J. Obst. & Gynec. 101:171, 1968.
15. May, H. C.: Carcinoma in situ of the vagina subsequent to hysterectomy for carcinoma in situ of the cervix, Am. J. Obst. & Gynec. 76:807, 1958.
16. Moertel, C. G., Dockerty, M. B., and Baggenstoss, A. H.: Multiple primary neoplasms, Cancer 14:221, 1961.
17. Novak, E. R., and Woodruff, J. D.: *Gynecologic and Obstetric Pathology* (Philadelphia and London: W. B. Saunders Company, 1963).
18. Patten, S. F., Regan, J. W., Obenauf, M., and Ballard, L. A.: Postirradiation dysplasia of uterine cervix and vagina: an analytical study of the cells, Cancer 16:173, 1963.
19. Reagan, J. W.: Personal communication.
20. Rutledge, F.: Cancer of the vagina, Am. J. Obst. & Gynec. 97:635, 1967.
21. Terzano, G.: Does irradiation influence the karyopyknetic index? Acta cytol. 3:413, 1959.
22. von Haam, E., and Albery, R.: Recurrent carcinoma and the presence of radiation cell changes, Acta cytol. 3:415, 1959.
23. Wachtel, E.: A simple cytological test for cancer cure, Brit. M. J. 1:20, 1958.
24. Zimmer, T. S.: Late irradiation changes, Cancer 12:193, 1959.

CHAPTER 20

The Cytopathology of Certain Benign Findings That May Be Confused with Malignancy

Cells With Multinucleation

GIANT CELLS* seen in cervicovaginal smears may be classified as follows in Table 20-1[7]:

Numerous other pathologic conditions of the female genital tract are associated with giant cells that do not ordinarily appear in cytologic material; the lesions are primarily in subepithelial locations, e.g., specific infectious granulomas.

HISTIOCYTES

Histiocytes in smears may appear singly or in groupings, as small clusters or in syncytia. Whether arranged singly or grouped, nuclei of individual histiocytic cells show similar characteristics. Nuclei have a mean size of about 41 μ^2; they are round to elliptical, at times with an indentation along one side and have finely dispersed chromatin. Small, single or double nucleoli are very commonly seen. At times, when histiocytes are secondary to an inflammatory process, the nuclear chromatin may appear more dense and mitotic activity can be readily observed.

*Syncytial giant cells are multinucleated cells having a common cytoplasm. By contrast, clustered cells, though closely apposed, have recognizable cytoplasmic borders.

TABLE 20-1.—CLASSIFICATION OF SYNCYTIAL GIANT CELLS SEEN IN CERVICOVAGINAL CYTOLOGY

A. Histiocytes
B. Benign endocervical cells
C. Viral inclusion cells—primarily herpes simplex (possibly other conditions such as condyloma acuminatum)
D. Trophoblast
E. Granulation tissue
F. Radiation or cellular alterations simulating radiation changes due to drug therapy.
G. Cells associated with megaloblastic anemias.
H. Malignant tumors

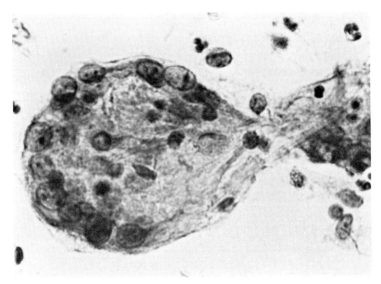

Fig. 20-1. – A giant histiocyte, closely apposed to suture material, from the vaginal smear of a 68-year-old woman who had a hysterectomy for carcinoma in situ of the cervix 2 months previously.

Only rarely do histiocytes form giant syncytia. In such instances, they are associated with a foreign body such as suture. The cells may contain up to a hundred or more nuclei (Fig. 20-1).

Singly occurring histiocytes may be confused with small malignant cells. The latter can be differentiated from histiocytes by their larger size, more irregular nuclei with heavier blocks of chromatin and less frequent nucleoli. Giant histiocytes and giant endocervical cells, described in the following section, offer a distinct problem in differential diagnosis.

Endocervical Cells

A sequel to chronic inflammatory disease of the cervix may be the formation of giant syncytial endocervical cells (Fig. 20-2, A). They are more common than are giant histiocytes. Endocervical cells rarely contain as many nuclei as giant histiocytes; in addition, giant endocervical cells have significantly larger nuclei than do histiocytes (Fig. 20-2, B). Table 20-2 compares salient features of giant endocervicals and giant histiocytes.

Giant endocervical cells can usually be readily differentiated from cells of endocervical adenocarcinoma. Giant endocervical cells rarely show cannibalism of leukocytes, a finding common to adenocarcinoma cells. While endocervical adenocarcinoma cells may occur as syncytia, such a grouping is not as characteristically observed as it is with giant endocervical cells. Adenocarcinoma cells are generally arranged in

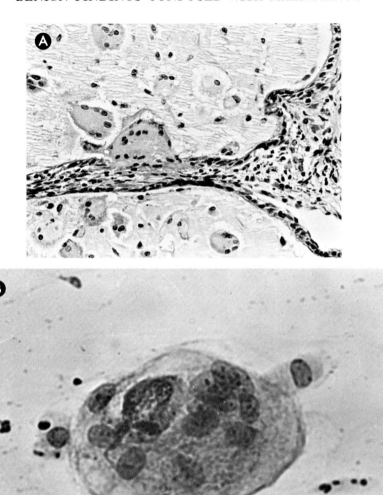

Fig. 20-2. — Giant endocervical cells. **A,** origin of the cells from the lining epithelium of endocervical glands (or clefts). Note the giant cells lying free in the gland lumina. **B,** a cell grouping. These cells rarely contain as many nuclei or have nuclei as small as those in giant histiocytes.

TABLE 20-2.—SALIENT COMPARATIVE CYTOLOGIC FEATURES OF GIANT ENDOCERVICAL
CELLS AND GIANT HISTIOCYTES

	GIANT ENDOCERVICALS	GIANT HISTIOCYTES
Nuclear size	Larger	Smaller
Number of nuclei	5–15	Up to hundreds
Nuclear chromatin pattern	Remarkably similar	Remarkably similar
Cytoplasmic staining	Pink	Gray to colorless
Exogenous cytoplasmic inclusions	Rare	Common
Occurrence	Fairly common	Rarely seen
Origin	From epithelium of endocervical columnar cells.	From syncytial replication of histiocytes from cervical stroma.

[From Tweeddale, D. N., *et al.*: Acta cytol. 12:298, 1968.]

more sharply outlined groupings than are cells representative of inflammatory processes. Nuclear findings are of paramount importance in differentiation; chromatin clumping and prominent nucleoli in cells of adenocarcinoma contrast sharply with finely granular chromatin and small, regular nucleoli in giant endocervical cells. Nuclei occupy a greater mean cell area in adenocarcinoma than in giant endocervical cells. In addition, the cytoplasm usually is eosinophilic in giant endocervical cells and cyanophilic in cells of adenocarcinoma.

VIRAL INCLUSION CELLS

Herpes simplex cervicovaginalis is the condition in which cells are most commonly associated with viral inclusions. Herpetic syncytial cells, similar in size to giant endocervical cells, contain 2–15 nuclei. The most salient morphologic hallmark of the former cell is the nuclear structure. Nuclei are enlarged and show either: 1) a few, small, vari-

Fig. 20-3.—Giant cells representative of infection by herpes simplex virus. **A,** the centrally placed large intranuclear inclusion is surrounded by a clear zone bounded by the nuclear membrane. The cytoplasm is indistinct. **B,** in this cell the nuclear chromatinic material is homogeneous, presenting a ground-glass picture. This nuclear pattern is commoner than that in **A.**

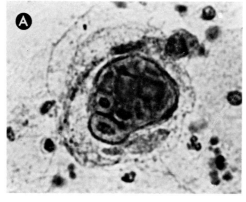
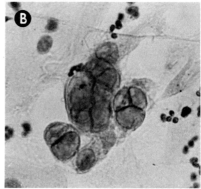

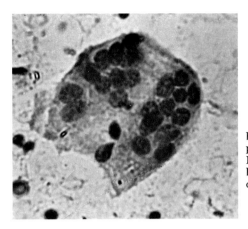

Fig. 20-4. – A syncytiotropho-blast giant cell from a touch preparation of the placenta. Notice the multiple heavy blocks of intranuclear chromatin.

ously sized clumps of chromatinic material, 2) a homogeneous, gray, ground-glass appearance or 3) an almost centrally placed acidophilic inclusion which occupies about half of its area and is surrounded by a clear zone. The cells are quite unlike those of adenocarcinoma. The latter cells have larger nuclei with characteristic malignant structure; nucleoli, though prominent at times, are not as large as herpetic inclusions. Because herpetic lesions are usually ulcerative, accompanying squamous cells may show changes characteristic of healing. Herpes infection does not guarantee the absence of carcinoma; indeed cancer is more likely to coexist.

Trophoblast

Cells of syncytiotrophoblast are rarely encountered in cytologic smears. They are most commonly observed in smears from patients with placenta praevia and during or following an abortion or delivery. Cell morphology is distinctive due to the nucleus which contains 10 to 12 heavy blocks of heavy chromatin, irregularly dispersed (Fig. 20-4). Nucleoli are not seen and this finding, combined with abundant cytoplasm, facilitates their differentiation from benign or malignant glandular epithelium.

Granulation Tissue

Fragments of granulation tissue may appear in cytologic preparations that are collected following a surgical procedure. They are represented by fairly large, irregular or oblong syncytia of fibroblastic cells with scattered inflammatory elements (Fig. 20-5). Such cell groupings are seldom confused with malignancy as nuclear characteristics of malignancy are not present. In fact, structure of the entire mass is often indistinct, due to cellular degeneration.

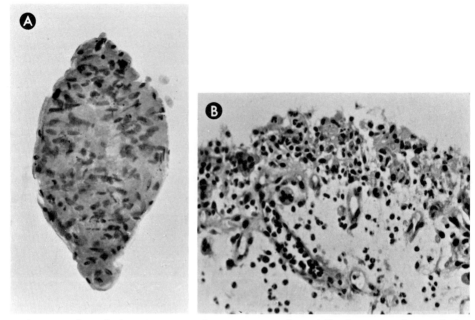

Fig. 20-5.—Granulation tissue. **A**, a large segment of partially degenerated granulation tissue in a vaginal smear taken several weeks after a hysterectomy. **B**, a histologic section from the patient whose cytology is shown in **A**. The surface granulation tissue is partly degenerated and represents the area from which the granulation bud shown in **A** originated.

Radiation, Cellular Alterations Due to Drug Therapy that Simulate Radiation Changes and Changes in Megaloblastic Anemias

Cellular changes incident to radiation therapy have been described in another section. Other conditions, such as folic acid deficiency, may be associated with cells showing remarkable morphologic similarity to those observed following radiation therapy. Administration of certain drugs (busulfan [Myleran] and possibly 5-Fluorouracil) has sometimes been associated with appearance of multinucleated cells, although changes resembling dysplasia are noted more frequently.

Malignant Tumors

Syncytial masses of tumor cells are characteristically observed in cytologic smears from patients with invasive cancer and, less frequently, from those with dysplasia. In other words, the presence of syncytial tumor cells may be correlated directly with the severity of the neoplastic process. On the other hand, syncytial cells may be components of a number of benign conditions (see above). In those instances, the most pertinent diagnostic feature is a benign nuclear structure. Cells associated with repair commonly occur in large sheets but seldom as large

TABLE 20-3.—CLASSIFICATION OF SPINDLE-SHAPED
CELLS SEEN IN CERVICOVAGINAL SMEARS

A. Epithelial origin	B. Stromal origin
1. Squamous	1. Smooth muscle
a. Benign	a. Benign
b. Malignant	b. Malignant
2. Glandular	2. Fibrous tissue
a. Benign	a. Benign
b. Malignant	b. Malignant

syncytial masses. The cells are often large with prominent nucleoli, appearing ominous at first glance. They are described in more detail on this page and the following two pages.

Cells of Elongated Appearance

Spindle-shaped cells, appearing singly or in sheets, are at least three times longer than they are wide. They may appear in cancerous or non-cancerous states and originate from either epithelium or connective tissue, usually the former. They are more commonly observed in benign than in malignant conditions. Epithelial spindle-shaped cells may represent benign or malignant squamous or glandular elements. Fibroblastic cells comprise the stromal spindle cells; the latter are seldom, if ever, representative of malignancy (see Table 20-3).

EPITHELIAL ORIGIN

Squamous

BENIGN.—Spindle-shaped squamoid cells have been described in smears of 2.2% of women with infections and in 1.9% of those without evidence of infection.[6] Cells appearing spindle shaped in smears reflect either growth characteristics in tissue or distortion created by trauma. In infectious processes, particularly ulcerations, elongated cells in smears result from growth patterns in tissue wherein regenerating cells elongate and flatten to cover a denuded surface (Fig. 20-6, *A* and *B*). Under such circumstances, surface cells may flatten as a result of pressures from accelerated growth of underlying cells and intraluminal pressure in the endocervical canal. Trauma may play a positive role in creating cell elongation. For example, smears taken in the early postpartum period may contain markedly elongated cells (Fig. 20-6, *C*). It is possible that some of the cells seen in postpartum smears arise from the stroma, but we believe that most originate from distorted squamous epithelium. Cells may also elongate if excessive pressure is exerted when a fresh smear is obtained.

The appearance of such cells is variable. The length/width ratio is at

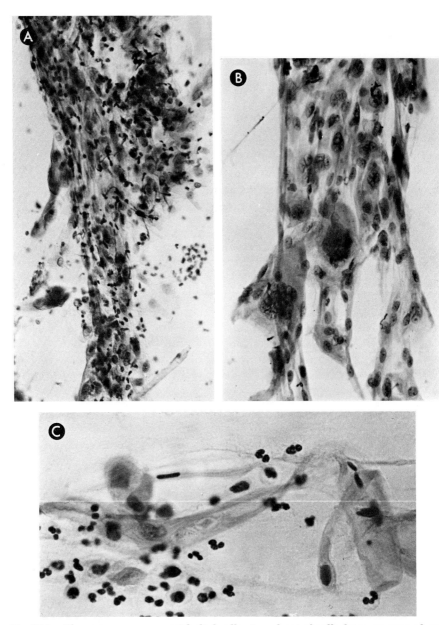

Fig. 20-6. — Elongate squamous epithelial cells. **A,** a sheet of cells from an area of repair. **B,** cells from repair following radiotherapy. Many are multinucleated. Squamous epithelial cells commonly appear spindled in smears taken after radiation therapy. **C,** distorted benign squamous epithelial cells in a smear taken 2 days post partum.

least 3:1 but may be as great as 50:1. The cytoplasm usually tapers gently to a point at each end. Cytoplasmic staining may be either acidophilic or cyanophilic. An almost centrally placed nucleus is regular in shape and elliptical, with a chromatin pattern that is characteristically benign. Nucleoli are only observed when such cells are associated with a healing process and are particularly prominent in cells regenerating after radiotherapy.

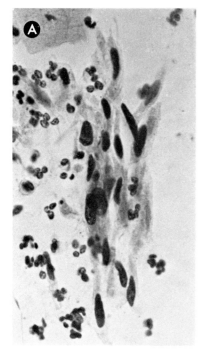

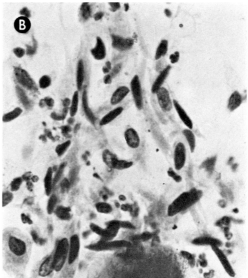

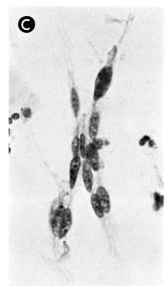

Fig. 20-7. — Malignant fiber cells. **A** and **B**, cells in a smear from a patient with in situ cancer of the cervix. **C**, cells in a smear from a patient with invasive squamous cell cancer of the cervix.

MALIGNANT. — As indicated previously, elongated cells in smears occur in direct proportion to the severity of the cellular alteration. For example, Reagan noted the spindle-cell population to be 1.5% in dysplasia, 1.8% in carcinoma in situ and 15% in invasive cancer.[4, 5] Others[1, 2, 3] have found the frequency of spindled cells, whether from in situ or invasive cancer, to be considerably greater (Fig. 20-7, A and B). Elongated cells are more common in smears from invasive keratinizing squamous cancer than in any other type of squamous neoplasm (Fig. 20-7, C). Cellular characteristics of malignant spindle cells have been described previously. In essence, they resemble benign spindle cells, save for malignant nuclear alterations. Cytoplasmic staining is variable: usually cyanophilic with in situ cancer and often eosinophilic with invasive cancer.

The shape of such cells may result from surface (juxtaluminal) flattening due to the pressure of growth from below and intraluminal pressure within the endocervical canal above, especially in cases of in situ cancer. Cells of invasive cancer have a tendency to grow in whorls containing flattened cells, probably reflecting the pressure of surrounding tissues. This is particularly true with keratinizing cancer.

The rare "tadpole" cell is almost never seen in a smear unless there is an underlying pathologic state. As in the case of spindle-shaped cells, prevalence of tadpole cells is proportional to the severity of malignancy; they are rarely observed in inflammatory conditions.

Glandular

BENIGN. — Glandular epithelium, whether benign or malignant, has a distinct tendency to form circumscribed groupings; therefore, spindling usually results from trauma. Cytoplasm of spindled glandular cells may be cyanophilic or acidophilic. Cells are often arranged in sheets in a palaside pattern. Nuclei, in contrast with those of spindled squamous cells, are eccentric rather than centrally located. The nucleus does not distort the cell outline and has a benign appearance. Endocervical cells following radiotherapy are not only of large size, with other signs of radiation effect, but are often irregular and elongated.

MALIGNANT. — Malignant glandular epithelium only rarely shows spindling in smears, and then probably reflects trauma incident to making the smear.

STROMAL ORIGIN

Smooth Muscle

BENIGN. — The elongated shape of the cells and benign, centrally placed ellipsoidal nuclei with scattered, fine chromatin structure permits their differentiation from spindled squamous cells in most instances.

MALIGNANT. — Cells of leiomyosarcoma are described on page 193. At times, such cells may be mistaken for spindled cells of squamous cell carcinoma. However, cells of squamous cancer only rarely have cytoplasmic processes as long as those of leiomyosarcoma.

Fibrous tissue

BENIGN.—Smears with fibroblasts are obtained most commonly following a recent operative procedure in the area from which the smear

Fig. 20-8.—Fibroblasts. **A,** smear from a patient with a vaginal ulcer following a hysterectomy. Note the prominent nucleoli. **B,** partially degenerated fibroblasts in a smear from the same patient as **A.** The cells have swollen and contain eosinophilic cytoplasm and indistinct nuclei. **C,** histologic section from the patients whose smears are shown in **A** and **B.** Note the spindled fibroblasts on the surface of the biopsy tissue.

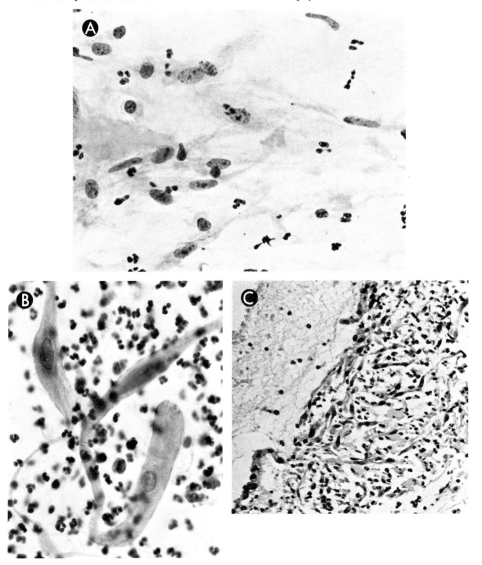

was taken. Less frequently, smears from primary ulcerative cervicovaginal processes may contain fibroblasts.

Fibroblasts are markedly elongated cells with pale or colorless, often indistinct, cytoplasm. The long cytoplasmic processes commonly cross over one another. (Fig. 20-8, *A*). At times, the cytoplasm may be swollen and stain an acidophilic color, possibly as a result of degeneration (Fig. 20-8, *B* and *C*). Centrally placed nuclei seldom distort the cell outline. The nuclear chromatin pattern is fine, and widely dispersed chromatin particles create a vesicular appearance. Single or double, small, regular nucleoli are constant findings.

MALIGNANT. — Endometrial stromal fibromyxosarcoma, a rare neoplasm, is characterized by malignant spindle-shaped cells with malignant nuclei and long cytoplasmic processes.

Cells of Large Size

A good general rule is that the larger the cell, the less the probability that it is malignant. For example, the following can be considered common conditions in which large cells are most likely to be seen: after radiation therapy; in repair; following parturition; in dry smears; following busulfan (Myleran) therapy; in megaloblastic anemias and in dysplasia.

FOLLOWING RADIOTHERAPY. — After radiotherapy, benign or malignant cells in smears predictably manifest a radiation reaction (RR). No other condition is so consistently accompanied by cells of increased size. Characteristics of these cells have been described in Chapter 19 and are shown in Figure 20-9.

WITH REPAIR. — Cells exfoliated from areas of repair are usually large, because they tend to spread and cover zones of ulceration and are occasionally tetraploid. In smears, the often irregular cells appear singly or in small groupings which may be syncytial. The cytoplasm is ordinarily eosinophilic; nuclei are round or elliptical with either a regular or irregular outline. While such nuclei are distinctly larger than those of normal cells, the nuclear/cytoplasmic ratio is not abnormally increased. The nuclei sometimes contain one or two nucleoli; the chromatin pattern is often vesicular so that close inspection readily detects benignity (Fig. 20-10).

Following radiotherapy, epithelial regenerating cells generally appear in large, clustered sheets. Individual cells are large and polygonal and contain a light cyanophilic cytoplasm. The nuclei contain finely dispersed chromatin and, almost always, a single, prominent nucleolus. In view of the small nuclear/cytoplasmic ratio, such cells should seldom be confused with malignant cells.

FOLLOWING PARTURITION. — Smears taken in the first few days follow-

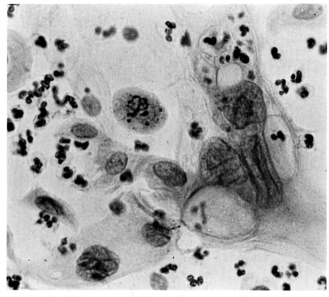

Fig. 20-9. – Large cells following radiotherapy. A group of large, benign cells with large, syncytially arranged nuclei and prominent cytoplasmic vacuoles. The patient had received radiotherapy for squamous cancer of the cervix.

Fig. 20-10. – Large cells in smears from a patient with a benign cervical ulcer. Such cells may be mistaken for those representing dysplasia (compare with Fig. 20-13).

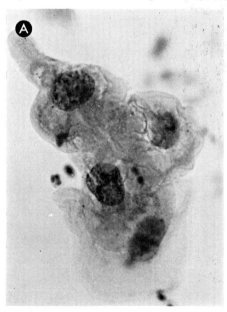

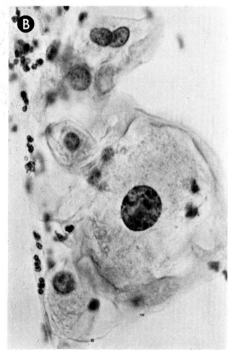

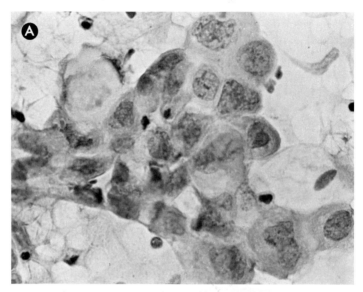

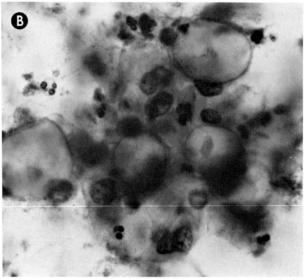

Fig. 20-11.—Large cells following parturition. **A,** a group of markedly enlarged, slightly degenerated gland cells in a smear from a woman who was 2 days postpartum. **B,** a group of postpartum gland cells containing large mucous vesicles.

ing childbirth may contain a variety of unusual cells. Spindled squamous elements have been described. Erythrocytes in varying states of preservation, cells from the placenta or decidua, endocervical glandular elements and unrecognizable degenerated cells are also seen. Endocervical cells often appear in large, slightly irregular sheets (Fig. 20-11, *A*). The individual cells may be many times larger than normal endocervical cells. The cytoplasm is eosinophilic and may contain large mucin-filled vacuoles (Fig. 20-11, *B*). Nuclei are enlarged in proportion to total cell size; they contain chromatin dispersed into large, swollen blocks separated by vesicular areas, and a fairly large, regular central nucleolus. The cellular changes probably result from traumatic dislocation of endocervical epithelium during delivery with subsequent degenerative changes.

IN DRY SMEARS. – If slides are not placed promptly into fixative after smears are made, or if no fixative is used, cells appear much larger than with prompt fixation. Inadequate fixation results in a uniform enlargement of the entire cell. However, staining characteristics, particularly of the nucleus, are less than optimal. Such changes are seldom confused with malignancy.

FOLLOWING BUSULFAN (MYLERAN) THERAPY. – Enlargement and, at times, multinucleation of cells after therapy with busulfan (Myleran) may occur (Fig. 20-12). Such therapy is more commonly followed by cellular changes resembling dysplasia.

Fig. 20-12. – Enlarged cells following Myleran therapy. **A** and **B**, sheets of cells which are markedly enlarged and have great similarity to cells representing spontaneous dysplasia. **C**, biopsy of the cervix of the patient whose cells are shown in **A** and **B** which evidences the Myleran change.

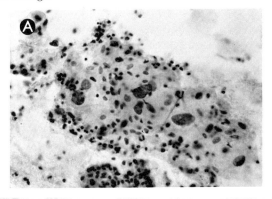

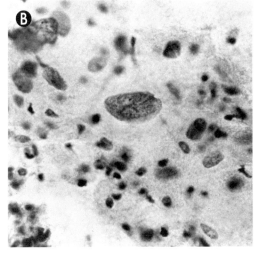

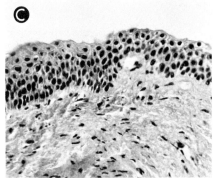

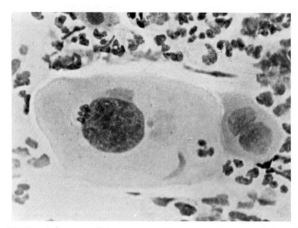

Fig. 20-13.—A large cell in a smear from a patient with dysplasia.

IN PERNICIOUS ANEMIA AND FOLIC ACID DEFICIENCY.—Some cells from patients with megaloblastic anemias may closely resemble those observed following radiotherapy.

IN DYSPLASIA.—At times, very large cells are observed in smears from patients with dysplasia (Fig. 20-13). Ordinarily, dysplastic cells are of predictable size and are several times larger than cells of in situ cancer. Only rarely are cells from in situ or invasive neoplasia as large as those described in the above sections.

Cells With Prominent Nucleoli

FOLLOWING RADIOTHERAPY.—During and immediately following radiotherapy, endocervical cells show the characteristics described on page 230. In addition, nucleoli may enlarge in the same proportion as other parts of the cell. Nucleoli are also prominent in regenerating epithelium following radiotherapy (Fig. 20-14). These changes should cause little confusion with malignancy, since other cell components are benign.

IN DECIDUA.—Decidual cells are seldom identified in cytologic smears. These cells are variable in size and generally polyhedral in shape. The cytoplasm stains lightly cyanophilic and may or may not contain small vacuoles. The nucleus is generally elliptical and may be irregular. Chromatin is finely dispersed, similar to that for dysplastic cells. However, the nucleus almost constantly contains a single, prominent nucleolus (Fig. 20-15). Because the nucleus/cytoplasmic ratio is small, a diagnosis of malignancy should not be entertained. The cells are similar to those associated with repair.

IN REPAIR.—These cells have been described above.

"INCLUSIONS".—These cells have been described above.

IN NEOPLASIA.—In general, increasing severity of squamous cancer is

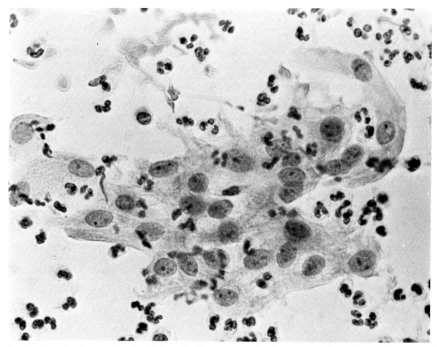

Fig. 20-14.—A sheet of spindled cells from a vaginal smear taken following radiation therapy. Such cells characteristically have prominent nucleoli and probably represent cells engaged in repair.

Fig. 20-15.—Cells of decidua from a touch preparation of endometrium in a pregnant uterus. Nucleoli are very prominent in smears stained by Papanicolaou's method but are not as easily observed in conventional histologic sections stained by hematoxylin and eosin.

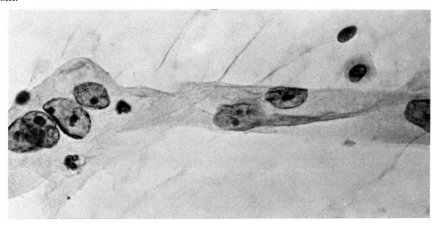

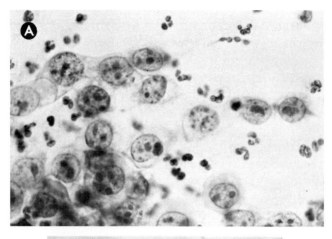

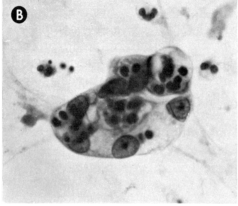

Fig. 20-16.—Prominent nucleoli in neoplasia. **A**, cells in a smear from a patient with invasive squamous cancer of the cervix. These large nonkeratinizing cells commonly contain nucleoli. **B**, a group of malignant cells from an endocervical adenocarcinoma. Adenocarcinoma cells invariably contain prominent nucleoli.

accompanied by a greater number of cells containing nucleoli. For example, nucleoli are absent in dysplastic cells but may be found in over 10% of those from invasive malignancy[4, 5] (Fig. 20-16, *A*). Nucleoli are constantly present in adenocarcinoma and become larger, more irregular and more frequently multiple with increasing degrees of malignancy (Fig. 20-16, *B*).

Notes on Hyperchromasia Associated With Blood and Cytology Following Cauterization

In the presence of significant quantities of blood, there is a tendency for the nuclear chromatin to stain with enhanced intensity. It is wise to use conservatism in evaluating such preparations, particularly in interpreting glandular cells.

Cautery to the cervix should not be applied prior to obtaining a cytologic smear. Cells are often "cooked" and so distorted that cytologic examination is not only of little value, but is subject to "overdiagnosis." Nuclear and cytoplasmic distortion under such circumstances can lead to an erroneous cytodiagnosis of malignancy, as nuclei may swell and nuclear chromatin may become irregularly condensed.

REFERENCES

1. Boschann, H. W.: Are spindle-shaped squamoid cells suggestive of a distinct type of carcinoma or of a distinct degree of cellular maturity? Acta cytol. 2:272, 1958.
2. Campos, J. R. de C.: Occurrence of spindle-shaped squamoid cells in carcinoma in situ, Acta cytol. 2:252, 1958.
3. Graham, R.: Occurrence of spindle-shaped squamoid cells in invasive carcinoma, Acta cytol. 2:259, 1958.
4. Reagan, J. W., and Hamonic, M. J.: The cellular pathology in carcinoma in situ, Cancer 9:385, 1959.
5. Reagan, J. W., Hamonic, M. J., and Wentz, W. B.: Analytical study of the cells in cervical-squamous cancer, Lab. Invest. 6:241, 1957.
6. Terzano, G.: Occurrence of spindle-shaped squamoid cells in infections, Acta cytol. 2: 241, 1958.
7. Tweeddale, D. N., *et al.*: Giant cells in cervico-vaginal smears, Acta cytol. 12:298, 1968.

Index